EUREKA!
THE MOTHER CAUSE OF SCOLIOSIS:

AND HOME EXERCISES TO STOP THE PROGRESSION OF SCOLIOSIS AND EVEN REVERSE IT! FOR AGES 1-22

Indeed this is the major cause of all the abnormal spinal curves!

never delay or wait for a miracle for your scoliosis, start the scoliosis treatment with the right exercises when the abnormal curve of scoliosis is still small and easier to correct, right after the initial diagnosis is made.

Dr. s.elia

BAD POSTURAL HABITS AND THE

LACK OF EXERCISES WILL GIVE
YOU A CROOKED SPINE .
THE RIGHT EXERCISES WILL GIVE
YOU A STRONG, HEALTHY,
FLEXIBLE SPINE, GOOD HEALTH,
GOOD POSTURE AND NO
ABNORMAL SPINAL CURVES!!

.

IT IS TIME TO STOP THE EPIDEMIC OF
IDIOPATHIC SCOLIOSIS THAT   AFFLICTS
YOUNG KIDS AND TEENAGERS BY
REMOVING THE CAUSATIVE FACTORS OF
THE LUMBAR-SACRAL-ILIAC JOINTS
IMBALANCE AND MALFUNCTION, WITH
THE RIGHT SPINAL EXERCISES AS SOON
AS THE DIAGNOSIS WITH THE X-RAYS IS
MADE , WITHOUT ANY DELAYS OR
OBSERVATION PERIODS!

Specific spinal exercises for the prevention and reduction of idiopathic scoliosis in short S.A.F.E.T.R.I.S..

never delay or wait for a miracle for your scoliosis, start the scoliosis treatment with the right exercises when the abnormal curve of scoliosis is still small and easier to correct, right after the initial diagnosis is made.

Specific spinal exercises for the prevention and reduction of idiopathic scoliosis in short S.A.F.E.T.R.I.S..

S.A.F.E.T.R.I.S. SPINAL ACTIVE
FLEXION EXERCISES TO REDUCE
IDIOPATHIC SCOLIOSIS. These
exercises are easy to do in the privacy of
your home , even in your own bed
without any equipment. These exercises
are designed to remove the cause of the
idiopathic scoliosis and restore the
normal function of the spinal-lumbar-
sacral joints and in the process make the
spine stronger more flexible without any
abnormal curves!!

 Disclaimer:
N.B. these exercises are good for anyone that has a
spine, but are not intended for people with spinal
fractures, spinal pathology or had surgery with
fusion and rods in their spines. If that is your case
consult your doctor for proper diagnosis, treatments
and recommendations. It is advisable to consult

your doctor before starting any strenuous exercises . Kids should be supervised by their parents and never push them to do more exercises than they are capable of doing.
Dr. S. ELIA

Self published by Dr. S.Elia
with   Kindle Direct Publishing at   amazon.com

TAKE CARE OF YOUR SPINE,
IT IS THE BACKBONE OF GOOD HEALTH,
GOOD POSTURE AND GRACE

Never delay the treatment of scoliosis with the

"wait and see "approach. Start the scoliosis treatment with the right exercises when the abnormal curve of scoliosis is still small and easier to correct.

DR. S.ELIA

Dedication:

I dedicate this book to the millions of patients with idiopathic scoliosis that will do the spinal active flexion exercises to reduce the idiopathic scoliosis(

S.AF.E.T.R..I.S.) daily and they will turn their abnormal scoliotic spines into strong, healthy, and flexible spines without any abnormal spinal curves and in the process they will get a good posture that will be the envy of many!!! They will prove to themselves and the world that indeed
there is hope to beat scoliosis with
S.A.F.E.T.RI.S.
The spine is the backbone of good health , good posture and with the spinal active flexion exercises   to reduce idiopathic scoliosis ,they can reverse the scoliotic spine especially when the abnormal curve is still small and easier to reverse!

TAKE CARE OF YOUR SPINE,
IT IS THE BACKBONE OF GOOD HEALTH,
GOOD POSTURE AND SPLENDOR

TABLE OF CONTENTS

1) Prologue:

After years of studying, researching, examining and observing spinal conditions especially the abnormal curves of the spine, scoliosis, kyphosis and lordosis, I found that many patients got spinal problems from lifting, carrying heavy objects, bad posture, sitting and working in awkward positions, or just slouching on their favorite sofa watching television.

I used traction, taping, stretching, spinal supports and manipulation, trying to correct the abnormal curves…
I observed the Adam's test on many normal and abnormal spines and I observed athletes that exercise everyday to have strong healthy spines without any abnormal spinal curves and a good posture that is the envy of many.
I came to the conclusion that the best way to prevent and treat scoliosis is spinal exercises and the patient has to have the motivation, the will, desire and determination to exercise daily.
Only the patient can do the exercises, NOBODY else can do the exercises for them.
I realize that many patients do not have the time or expense to go to the gym every day or buy expensive equipment to use in their homes…
Therefore, I combined the observation of the Adam's test that a functional scoliosis straightens when the patient bends forwards, and similar exercises that professional athletes do daily to have a healthy, strong spines with no abnormal curves, to design the SPINAL ACTIVE FLEXION EXERCISES TO REDUCE IDIOPATHIC SCOLIOSIS, in short S.A.F.E.T.R.I.S.
The exercises are simple and easy to do in the privacy of their homes, even in their own bed without any equipment.
No need to go to the gym or any other excuse of no

time to exercise.

All they have to do is to do the exercises daily and their spine, posture and health will thank them.

The spine is the backbone of good health ,good posture and splendor. Take care of your precious spine for good health.

It is my strong belief that if everybody exercises daily with the S.A.F.E.T.R.I.S. exercises they will be rewarded handsomely with good health, good posture and no abnormal curves.

Although I designed these exercises for people with idiopathic scoliosis to stop the progression of their abnormal curve called scoliosis, If everyone, young and old start doing the S.A.F.E.T.R.I.S. Exercises daily, perhaps the idiopathic scoliosis will be eliminated, or at least greatly reduced in the near future!

Disclaimer:

N.B. these exercises are good for anyone that has a spine, but are not intended for people with spinal fractures, spinal pathology or had surgery with fusion and rods in their spines. If that is your case consult your doctor for proper diagnosis, treatments and recommendations. As a matter of fact you should consult your doctor before starting any

strenuous exercises . Kids should be supervised by their parents and never push them to do more exercises than they capable of doing.
Dr. S. ELIA

2)Introduction.

In my previous books, I wrote about the causes of idiopathic scoliosis and ways to prevent and treat scoliosis with exercises.

In this book I will write about the mother cause, in other words the major cause of idiopathic scoliosis and I will concentrate on the specific   spinal exercises S.A.F.E.T.R.I.S. and elaborate why these exercises are the best in stopping the progression of scoliosis. **By exercising daily the people with scoliosis will have a better chance to stop the progression of scoliosis and even reverse their scoliosis if that abnormal curve is small** .

 Without any exercises and bad postural habit's the scoliosis will get worse. Over a period of time, inflammation, irritation and arthritic changes will turn a small functional scoliosis into a structural scoliosis and a lifelong suffering. The purpose of the exercises is to stop the progression of the abnormal functional curve and prevent it from becoming a structural scoliosis with inflammation, irritation and arthritic changes and a life long suffering.

 People diagnosed with scoliosis know what scoliosis is by seeing the x-rays of their spines . Many of them they will be wondering what is idiopathic scoliosis ?. In simple words scoliosis means a crooked spine.

3) WHAT IS SCOLIOSIS?

Scoliosis is an abnormal sideways spinal curve to
the right or left side of the spine. They call it
idiopathic because they do not know what causes
that abnormal curve.

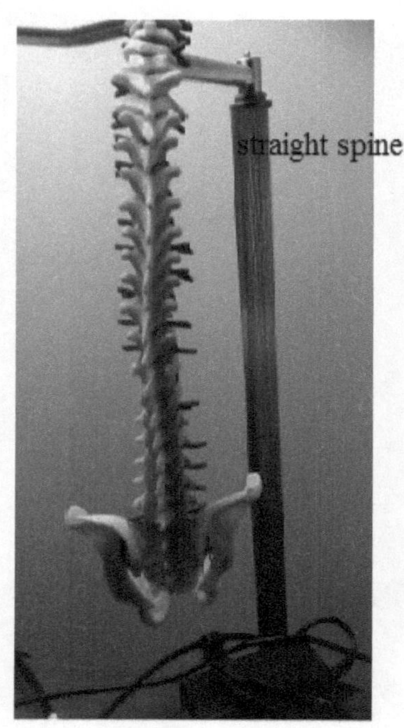

straight spine

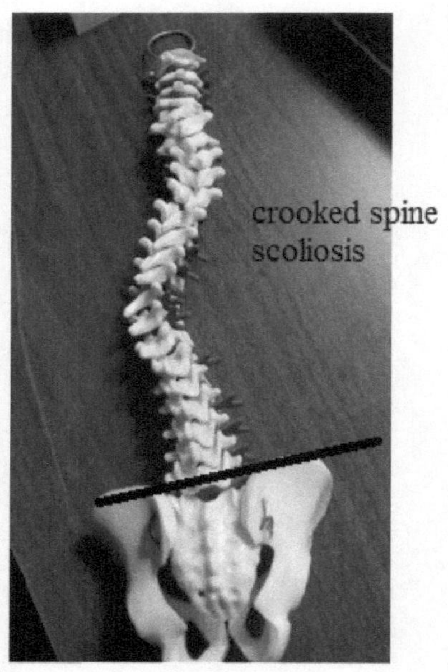

crooked spine
scoliosis

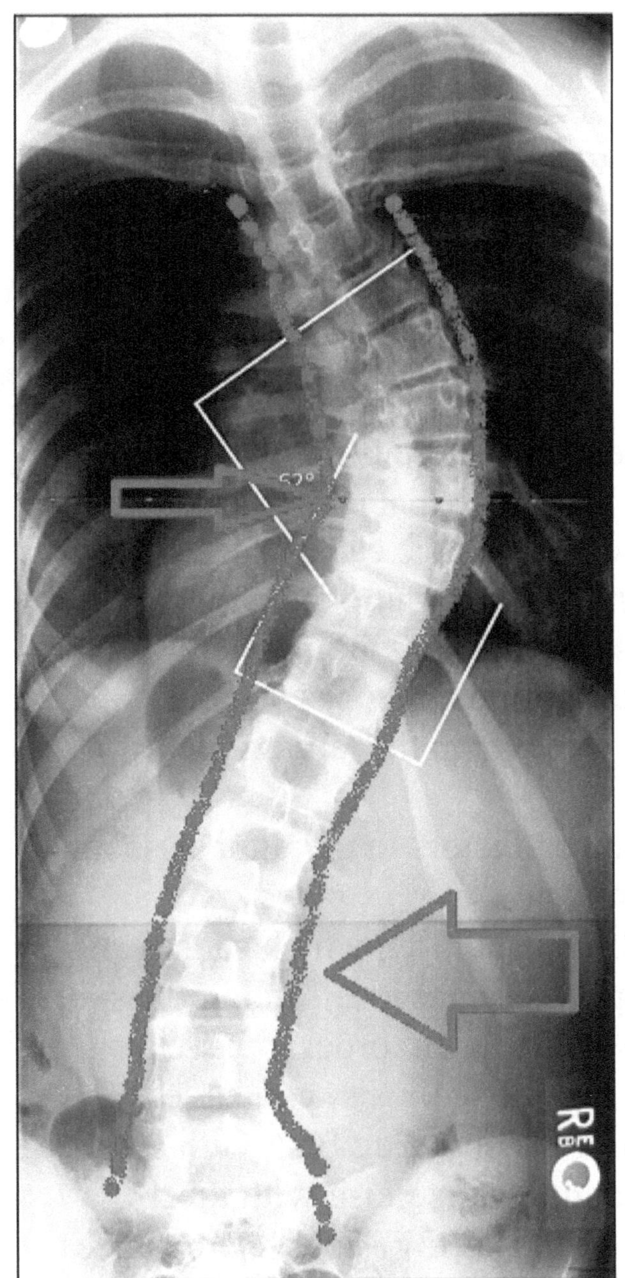
57°
R
E
B

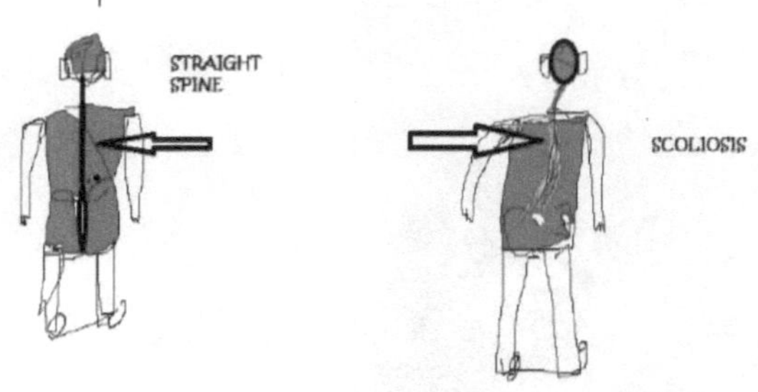

The fact that they call it idiopathic with no known cause does not mean that there is no causative factors that cause this abnormal curve. In my previous books I described the causes of the idiopathic scoliosis. As a matter of fact there are three major causes that cause an imbalance to the lumbar-sacral-Ilium joints, the base of the spine, forcing the spine to develop the abnormal sideways curve.

The three contributing factors to the lumbar-sacral-iliac imbalance are:

1) A true anatomical short leg which causes an imbalance to the pelvis sacral area forcing the spine to form a sideways curve . In order to have a correction of this type of scoliosis, you have to correct the length of the short leg first, with a heel lift or a shoe lift and then exercise with the S.A.F.E.T.R.I.S. exercises to restore the balance and normal function to the lumbar-sacral-iliac joints.

Fortunately with the elimination of poliomyelitis

with the polio vaccines not many people have a true anatomical short leg unless they had a leg fracture or other cause, but many people have a functional short leg due to a pelvic-sacral imbalance.

2)bad postural habits while sitting standing or walking causes an imbalance and strain to the pelvis-sacral-lumbar joints creating a functional short leg that creates the lumbar-sacrum-iliac imbalance whish is the perfect condition for the development of scoliosis.

3) injuries and strains, even by bending over to pick up a pen can cause a strain,   to the pelvis-sacral-lumbar spine joints creating the perfect conditions for the development of the abnormal curve called scoliosis.

<u>In other words the mother cause of scoliosis, or the causative factor of the idiopathic scoliosis is the imbalance of the pelvis-sacral-lumbar joints</u> caused by a short leg, bad postural habits and strains and injuries to the base of the spine creating the perfect conditions for the development of an initial abnormal curve at the lumbar spine area and a secondary compensatory abnormal curve to the thoracic spine due to the righting reflex trying to bring the centre of gravity within the body's base which are the sacrum and the feet.

See the diagram below of the mother of scoliosis and how the idiopathic scoliosis is formed over a period of time and eventually will cause inflammation, irritation , arthritic and structural changes.

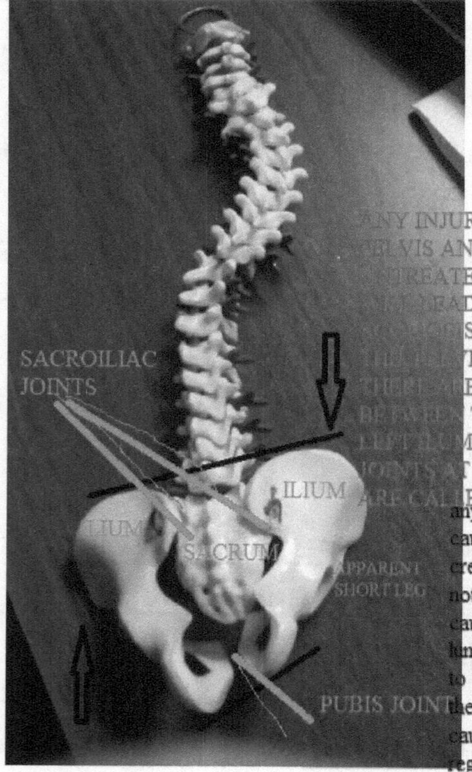

4) SIGNS AND SYMPTOMS OF SCOLIOSIS

People with scoliosis might have pain in the low back, neck and shoulder blades and sometimes in the early stages, the scoliosis can be without any pain.

When the scoliosis is severe with the spine severely crooked it can cause serious health problems affecting the lungs, heart and other the parts of the body .

People with scoliosis have uneven shoulders, one shoulder blade is more prominent than the other, and have a rib hump, One hip higher than the other uneven hips arms or leg lengths.

 Sometimes   other people, family friends and classmates notice the scoliosis first, for the obvious reason that people with scoliosis they cannot see their spine on their back, but others have a better view of others' spine.

5) DIAGNOSIS OF SCOLIOSIS

Anybody can see a crooked spine, but the proper
diagnosis of scoliosis is made with x-rays and
measuring the angle of the abnormal spinal curve
with the COBB method.   The angle
measurements is to see the degree of the abnormal
spinal curve. The greater the degree, the worse the
scoliosis curvature is.
A scoliosis is defined as a lateral spinal curvature
with a **Cobb** angle of 10° or more.

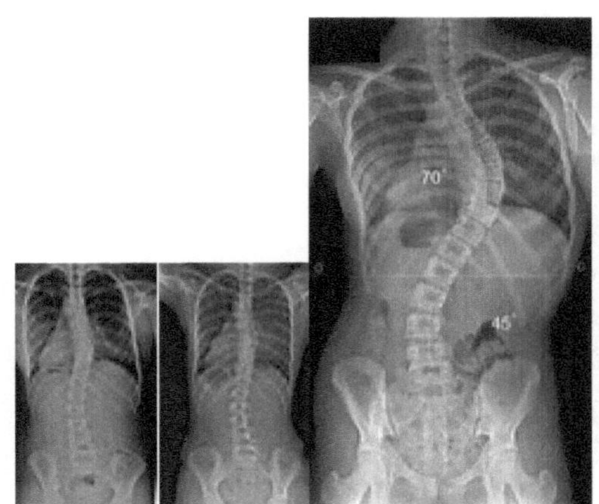
70°
45°

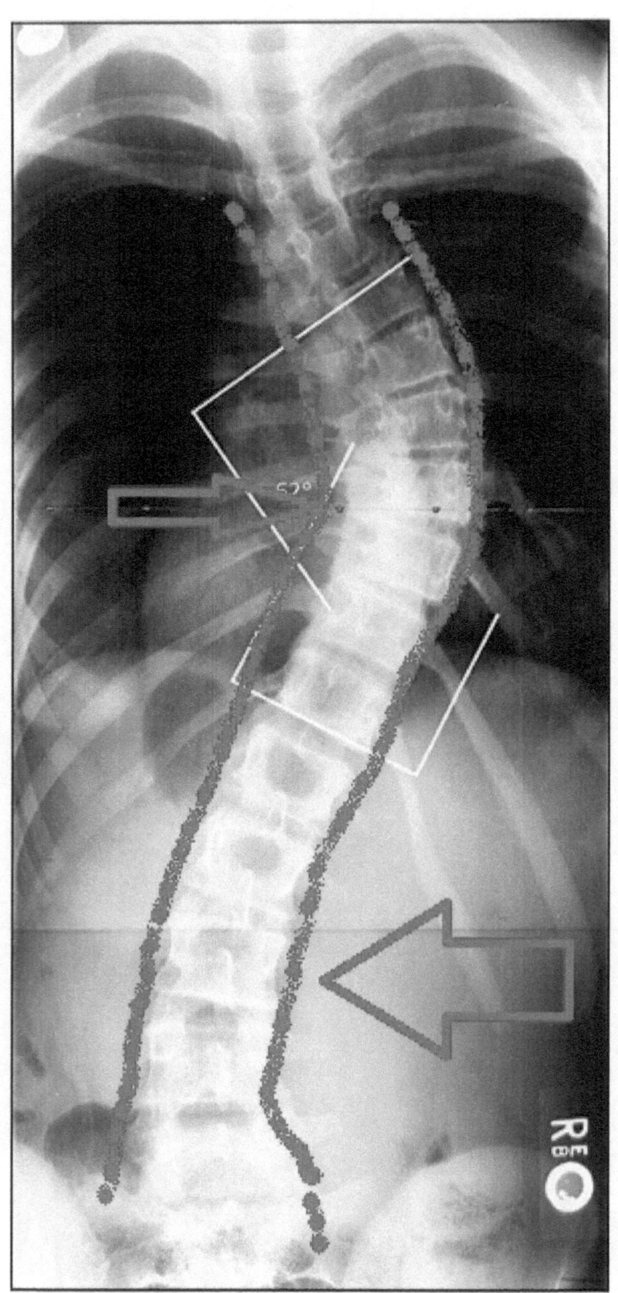

52°

6) TWO TYPES OF SCOLIOSIS

1) CONGENITAL   SCOLIOSIS DEVELOPED
BEFORE BIRTH

The congenital scoliosis is present before the baby
is born and it is developed while the baby was in
the mother's womb.
The congenital scoliosis is the worst type of
scoliosis and it is very difficult to treat. The bones
of the spine are usually malformed, fused together,
or half developed forming acute angles causing
severe abnormal spinal curves . This type of
scoliosis is treated by the specialist orthopedic and

neurosurgeons .

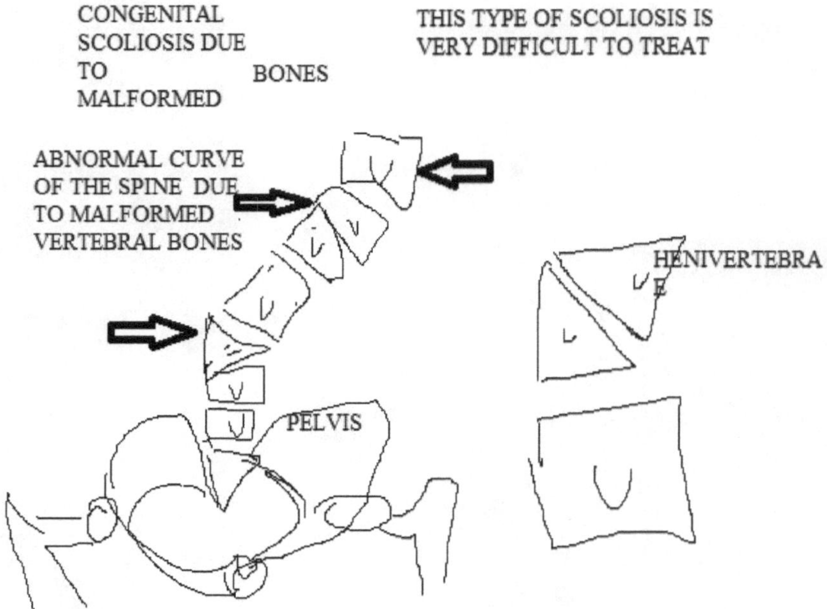

<u>The "mother cause" of congenital scoliosis is the malformed vertebral bones and hemi-vertebral bones that formed abnormal spinal curves that are difficult to treat.</u>

Any time we see malformed vertebral bones and hemi-vertebrae that cause an abnormal spinal curve we know that it is congenital scoliosis and that's treated by orthopedic doctors and neurologist. For years the scientific community was trying to find the cause of those malformed and distorted bones that were causing the **<u>mother cause of congenital scoliosis</u>** .

Fortunately their efforts and prayers were

answered by a research done in England that found the contributing factor to the malformed spinal bones.

<u>The contributing factor of " the mother cause of congenital scoliosis" is a nutritional deficiency of folic acid, also know as vitamin B9 one of the B vitamins.</u>
Folic acid received its name from the Latin word folium, meaning "foliage," because it is found in high concentrations in green leafy vegetables, such as spinach, kale, beet greens, and Swiss chard asparagus and other   fruits and vegetables.

For years the scientific community did not know the cause of the congenital scoliosis and they were doing the best they could to treat this abnormal spinal curve with observation, surgery, braces and exercises with limited success due to the severity of the abnormal curve.

  Thanks to the   research done by British scientists found that the causative factor for such abnormalities to the spine and other   deformities to the unborn baby, such as cleft palate and cleft lips, might be nutritional deficiencies during pregnancy such as folic acid .
And I quote from his published research: "We already know that **folic acid** reduces the risk of

NTD ,neural tube defects, including spinal bifida. Our research suggests that **folic acid** also helps **prevent** facial **clefts**, another common birth defect." Jan 26, 2007Allen J. Wilcox, M.D., Ph.D., lead NIEHS author on the new study published online in the *British Medical Journal*. "

His research suggest that other abnormalities of the spine , such as spinal bifida and spinal neural abnormalities will be prevented when the pregnant mothers take folic acid during their pregnancy. Thanks to the above research, the mother cause of congenital scoliosis is prevented , when the pregnant mothers take folic acid supplements during their pregnancy.

The folic acid SUPPLEMENTATION ,that prevents the contributing factor, THE LACK OF FOLIC ACID, to the mother of congenital scoliosis, is the ONE STITCH IN TIME TO PREVENT NINE.   When the mother takes folic acid , the one stitch in time, during her pregnancy, it prevents the mother of congenital scoliosis to develop, "the malformed spinal bones," thus saving nine stitches, i.e. the severe abnormal spinal curve of the congenital scoliosis.

 Now the doctors advice the pregnant women to take folic acid to prevent the   congenital scoliosis, neural tube deficiencies , cleft palate and cleft lips and perhaps other congenital abnormalities.

The recommended daily dietary allowance for folic

acid for adults is 400 micrograms or 0.4 mg. and all pregnant women should ask their doctor for nutritional advice and folic acid supplementations.

2) ACQUIRED SCOLIOSIS AFTER BIRTH

When the abnormal spinal curve develops after birth, then it is called acquired scoliosis,   has many causes and is classified according to the causative factor and the age of the patient:

1) Traumatic scoliosis, due to an injury to the spine causing the abnormal curve . Can occur at any time. it is an emergency and is treated in a hospital by the specialist.

2) pathological scoliosis due to some pathology on the spine, like tumors, fracture, infections, etc . can occur at any time and is treated in a hospital by specialists.

3)Degenerative scoliosis results from degenerative changes or collapsed vertebrae of the spine which usually is found in older people and treated by specialist.

4) neuromuscular scoliosis from abnormalities of the central nervous system or muscles disease, like cerebral palsy, muscular atrophy etc

The above four   types of scoliosis are best treated by the orthopedic specialist and neurologists and we will not discuss them any further in this book.

5) The Idiopathic scoliosis which apparently has no known cause, AT LEAST UP TO NOW, and occurs during the growing years of the youngsters. This is the type of scoliosis we will discuss in this book.

The idiopathic scoliosis is classified according to the age of the patient.

 A) infantile idiopathic scoliosis   ages 0 to 3 years old

B) juvenile idiopathic scoliosis ages 4 to 9

C) adolescent idiopathic scoliosis ages 9 to 20

D) adult idiopathic scoliosis when the

abnormal curve develops after age 20.

If the child was normal and free of any abnormal spinal curves at birth then there must be a real cause for that abnormal curve called idiopathic scoliosis , to develop. And that's what we are going to explore in this book, causes, diagnosis, prevention and treatments .

For too long the scientific community has been stuck with that   archaic name, idiopathic scoliosis, since the era of Hippocrates , meaning that they do not know the cause of the abnormal curve. The patients are not served well with that definition of idiopathic scoliosis which develops mostly during the growing years of the youngsters . When the doctors diagnose this type of scoliosis, they throw their hands up in the air saying , "we can not do anything about it, we do not know the cause" and "we will wait and see what happens in the future" and that's not good enough for the youngsters . Their spinal curve will get worse as time goes by wasting precious time with that advice.
Eventually they send them to an orthopedic specialist for evaluation, but by then the abnormal curve is getting worse requiring uncomfortable braces and surgery.

7) TWO TYPES OF IDIOPATHIC SCOLIOSIS

1) functional idiopathic scoliosis is an abnormal
spinal curve but all vertebral bodies and joints
appear normal without any changes. when the
Adam's bend forward test is performed the spine
straightens out. This type of scoliosis is a good
candidate for correction with   spinal active flexion
exercises to reverse scoliosis, in short
S.A.F.E.T.R.I.S.   when the bad postural habits are
also eliminated.
It is unlikely that a true short leg exist, but it might
be a functional short leg present due to a lumbar-
sacral-iliac imbalance, the mother cause of the
abnormal curve.

2) in structural scoliosis there are already structural and arthritic changes to the vertebral bodies and spinal joints with muscle spasm and rigidity. This is a long standing abnormal curve which started out as a functional scoliosis but without the proper treatments and exercises , ended up as a structural scoliosis. This type of scoliosis is difficult to treat and almost impossible to reverse. That is why it is very important to start the treatment with exercises without delay when the scoliosis is small   and easier to correct.
With the right exercises the structural scoliosis will improve the mobility and flexibility of the spine .

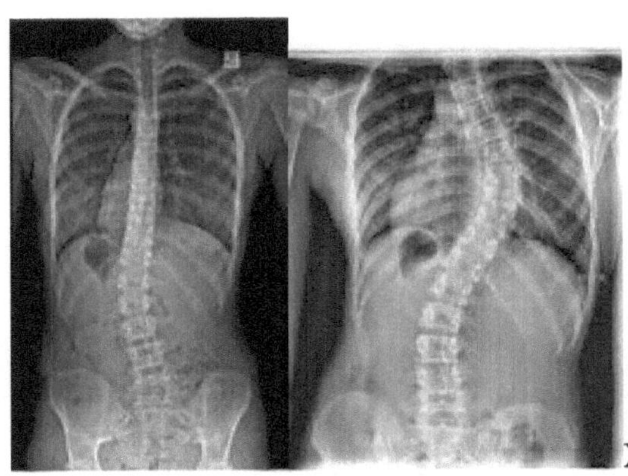

x-rays of functional idiopathic scoliosis still in the early stages of the abnormal spinal curves. These spines are good candidates for correction with the spinal active flexion exercises to reduce the idiopathic scoliosis

,provided that any bad postural habits are eliminated.

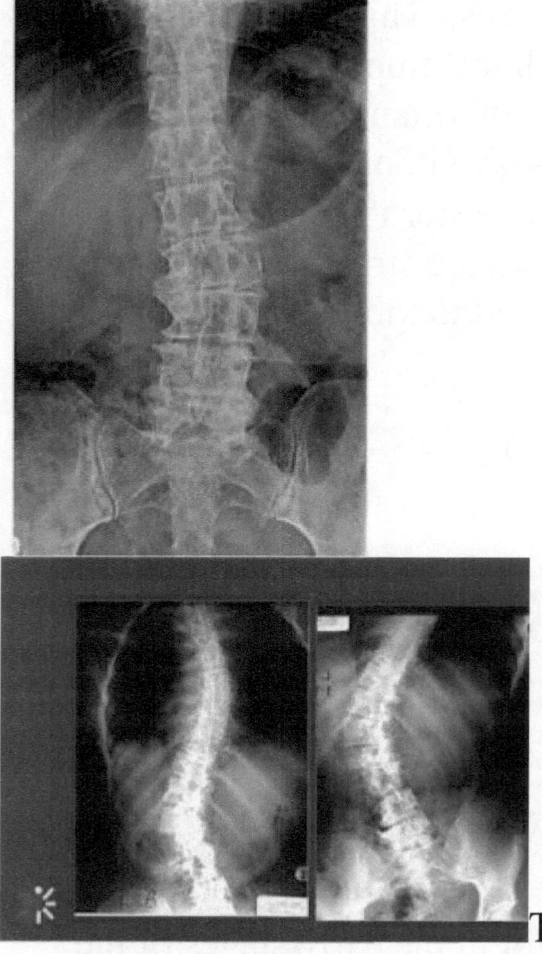

This is the structural idiopathic scoliosis with obvious structural and arthritic changes to the spinal joints in the lumbar vertebral joints . This is a long

lasting crooked spine with arthritic changes   and it
is very difficult to treat and almost impossible to
reverse. People with this type of structural
scoliosis can still exercise with the
S.A.F.E.T.R.I.S. exercises to increase the mobility
and flexibility of the spine and reduce the muscle
spasm that might be there. They should go easy on
the exercises and do all the exercises they can and
never strain themselves. It took a long time for this
condition to reach this stage and they should
expect miracles overnight.   That is why the
exercises and treatments should start as soon as
possible when the initial diagnosis is made. Any
delay causes inflammation and arthritic changes
and a lifelong suffering.

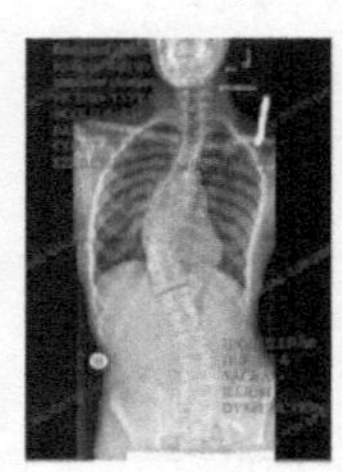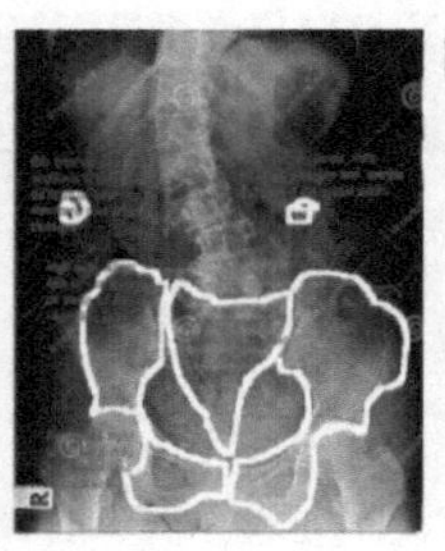

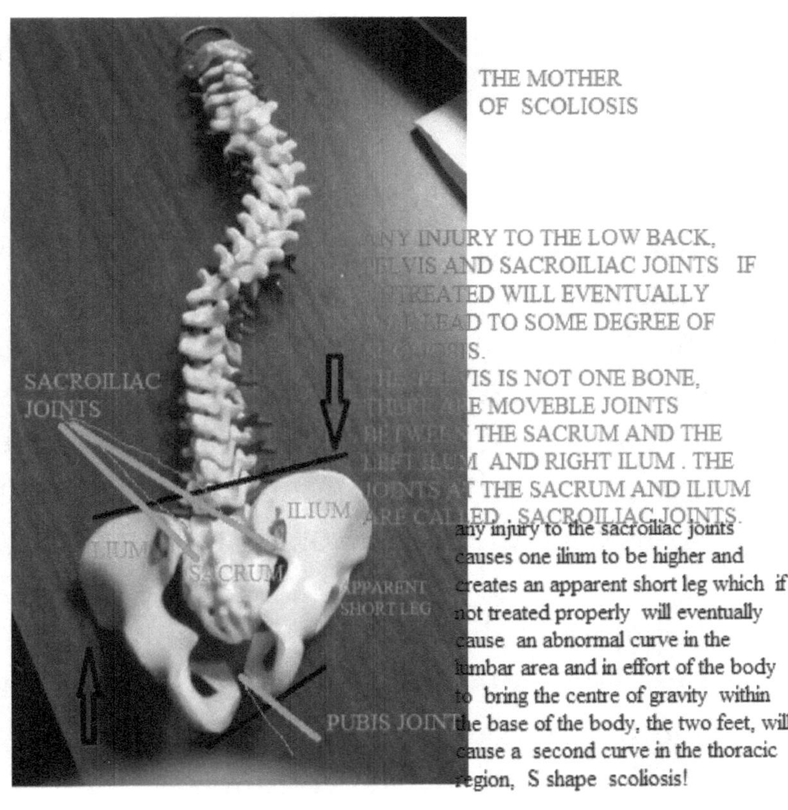

8) THE MOTHER CAUSE OF IDIOPATHIC SCOLIOSIS.

This is the million dollar question that baffles the medical and scientific community from time immemorial. What causes the abnormal curve of idiopathic scoliosis?.
Every year governments and other agencies spend

millions of dollars trying to unravel the mystery cause of this abnormal curve called idiopathic scoliosis. Every now and then they come up with these fancy theories as the cause of idiopathic scoliosis, but thank god they are only theories and not a fact. These theories are the figment of someone's vivid imagination . They blame heredity ,the genes, the DNA, selenium   and even that the bones grow faster than the spinal nerves forcing the spine into a scoliotic curve.!! I am just wondering what they will come up with next.

The idiopathic scoliosis is a structural problem affecting the structure, THE FRAME of the human body and in particular the spine where its base start at the lumbar-sacrum-ILIUM joints.

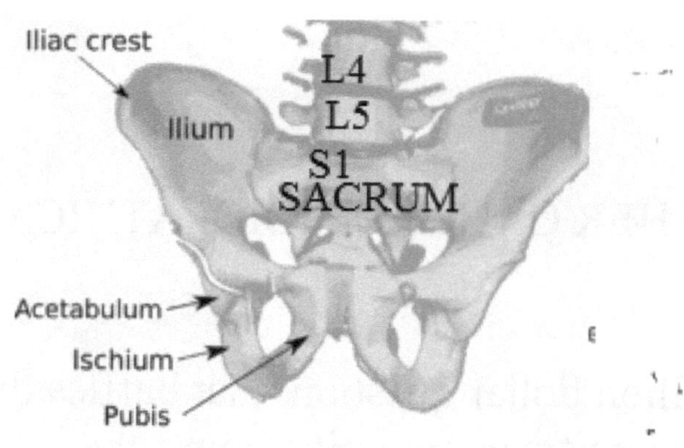

The human pelvis is not a rigid fused bone. It is

made up from the left and right Ilium(hip bones) joint with the sacrum in the middle to form the base, the foundation of spine. The sacrum is part of the spine with five distinct segments S1, S2, S3, S4 and S5 before is fused completely by the age of 18 or later. The sacrum plays a key role in supporting the upper body and connecting it to the lower body. From its position wedged between the hip bones, the sacrum stabilizes the entire pelvic girdle.. In this way, the sacrum acts much like a keystone in an arch, transferring the weight from the structure of the human body above and dispersing it out through the pelvis and into the legs below.

The pelvis is not fused but has functional joints at the sacrum-iliac joints and pubic joints. These joints have strong ligaments to hold them together but strains and sprains often happen to these joints to create the lumbar-sacral-iliac imbalance, the **MOTHER OF SCOLIOSIS**

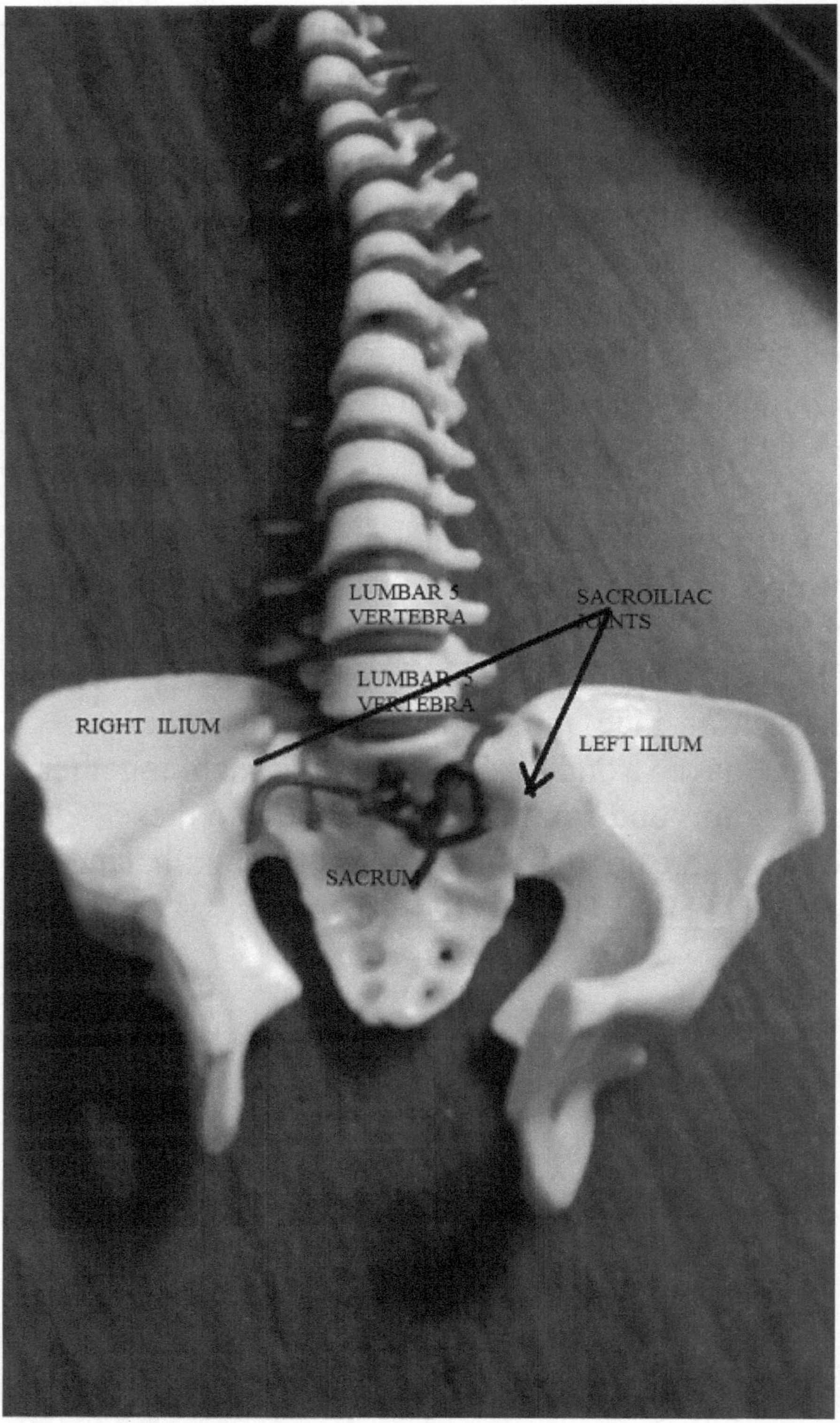

LUMBAR 5
VERTEBRA
SACROILIAC
JOINTS
LUMBAR 5
VERTEBRA
RIGHT ILIUM
LEFT ILIUM
SACRUM

When we look at any x-ray of the idiopathic scoliosis we always see, without exception, uneven pelvis, with one ileum higher than the other and the abnormal curve starting at the base of the spine the SACRUM, the holy bone, as the Greeks called it.

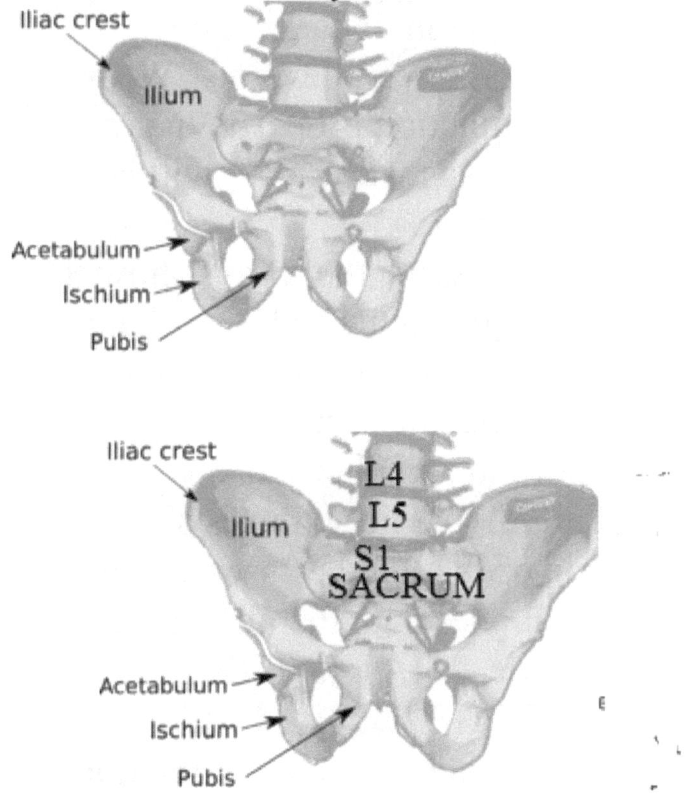

Why did they call the sacrum the holy bone?

<u>because of its major importance for the integrity of the human structure.</u> The sacrum joins the hipbones, the left and right Ilium at the sacroiliac joints and forms the base ,the foundation of the spine at the lumbar-sacral joints. From its position wedged between the hip bones, the sacrum stabilizes the entire pelvic girdle As long as the lumbar-sacrum-ileum joints are functioning properly and   are level and in balance, NO IDIOPATHIC SCOLIOSIS   can develop. When the above joints do not function properly, that's when the idiopathic scoliosis will start (will be born) at the base of the spine.

In a normal, non scoliotic spine the x-rays show the pelvic bones , left and right Ilium to be level and the sacrum sitting nicely between them and the spine sitting right on top of the sacrum without any deviation or any abnormal spinal curve.

Since the x-rays of all idiopathic scoliosis show an abnormal relationship of the lumbar-sacrum-pelvic bones with one Ilium higher than the other and the sacrum tilted to one side, THAT IS THE MOTHER CAUSE OF THE IDIOPATHIC SCOLIOSIS, it is the imbalance ,and dysfunction of the lumbar-sacrum-Ilium joints.

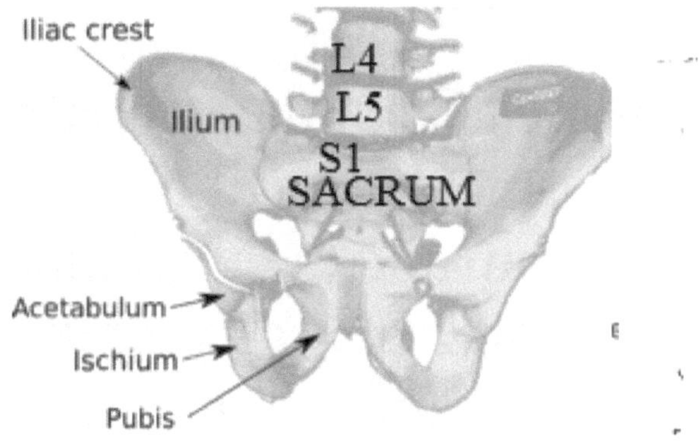

I

HIC

SCOLIOSIS

IDIOPAT

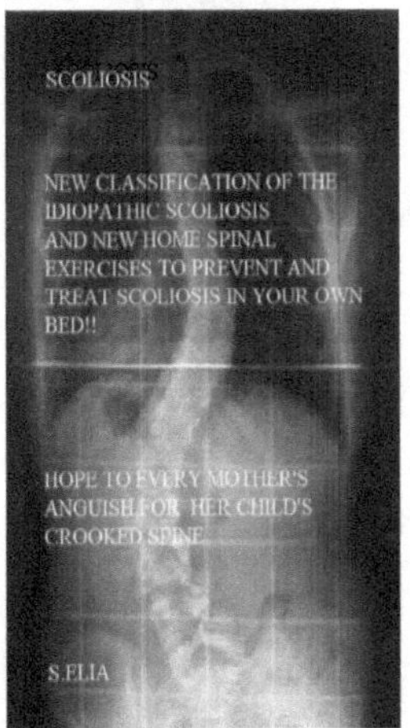

The MOTHER CAUSE , or in other words the major cause of the idiopathic scoliosis is the imbalance of the lumbar-sacral-Ilium and the malfunction of these joints , with the sacrum tilted to one side and one Ilium going higher, creating a functional short leg on that side and distorts the base of the spine, which is the sacrum with the pelvis. when that happens the spine is forced to follow the sacrum, which tilted to one side and forms an abnormal curve called scoliosis. The longer that imbalance AND MALFUNCTION remains, the bigger the abnormal curve will be. There are many contributing factors that can cause this lumbar-sacral-Ilium imbalance:
 1) a true anatomical short leg. that's the true short leg scoliosis. Forming the " true short leg scoliosis"
2) bad postural habits when sitting ,

walking, standing or working in an awkward position for too long. that includes the POSTURAL SCOLIOSIS and the POSITIONAL SCOLIOSIS of all ages, and that can include the NEUROMUSCULAR SCOLIOSIS types scoliosis, like the cerebral palsy , due to prolong sitting or lying in awkward positions.

3)lumbar-sacral straining or lifting accidents , sacroiliac joint straining or injuries, creating a functional short leg , forcing the sacrum to tilt to one side , forcing the spine to tilt and create an abnormal curve at the base of the spine.. That includes the BABYSITTING SCOLIOSIS in girls from straining the lumbar-sacral pelvic joints from lifting heavy babies, the POST-TRAUMATIC SCOLIOSIS of all ages, from lifting, falls or straining the lumbar-sacral area.

9) To conclude and summarize .

One might think that there are a lot of causes and names for the scoliosis, but in reality there can be condensed into only just three causes , or a combination of the **following three contributing factors that cause the lumbar-sacral-iliac imbalance, the mother of the so called idiopathic scoliosis.**

<u>1) postural scoliosis</u>, from poor habitual postural positions, when prolong sitting, standing or lying down as in the case of babies (positional infantile scoliosis) when they hold the babies and they put them to sleep on the same position. All these poor postural positions cause a lumbar-sacral-iliac joints strain and malfunction , creating the perfect condition for the MOTHER CAUSE OF SCOLIOSIS to be born and an abnormal curve to start with the classical x-ray findings.

<u>2) post-traumatic scoliosis</u>, from some sort of injury, strain or sprain in the low back , sacroiliac joints, from lifting or twisting, causing an apparent short leg , the lumbar-sacral-iliac imbalance, (the mother cause of scoliosis) and the creation of primary low back scoliosis and a secondary compensatory spinal curve in the thoracic area to compensate for the low back spinal curve. The secondary curve at the thoracic area is

the body's attempt to bring the centre of gravity within the base of the body the sacrum and , the two feet. That is the so called righting reflex. <u>The righting reflex, is a reflex that corrects the orientation of the body when it is taken out of its normal upright position.</u> or the centre of the body's gravity centre.

<u>3)   A true short leg scoliosis</u>, when there is a true short leg which causes an imbalance in the lumbar-sacral- pelvic region,(the mother of scoliosis) creating an abnormal lumbar area curve in the spine,   and a compensatory curve in the thoracic region. Again due to the righting reflex. That's it, just the three major contributor factors above, or a combination of the three causing the lumbar-sacral-iliac imbalance,(the mother of scoliosis) creating the perfect conditions for the abnormal spinal curve to develop . Any attempt to treat the so called idiopathic scoliosis, you have to correct or eliminate   the above three contributing factors first, in order to stop the progression of the abnormal curve, called scoliosis,

and even reverse it back to normal.
When the above contributing factors are
eliminated, and with the proper exercises, the
lumbar-sacral-iliac imbalance and malfunction will
return to normal and the abnormal curve will
reverse back to normal, especially when the
abnormal curve is small.

**<u>It is very important what precipitated
the lumbar-sacral-pelvic imbalance</u>**,
but what is the most   important thing is
**<u>to recognize that this lumbar-sacral-
Ilium imbalance and these joints
malfunction is "THE MOTHER
CAUSE" of every idiopathic scoliosis
and it is present on the x-rays of every
crooked spine.</u>**
What really matters is to **<u>recognize the
significance of this</u>** imbalance and
malfunction of these joints, **as a
causative factor of the idiopathic
scoliosis.** and try to correct it as soon
as possible , by eliminating the

precipitating factors that created the lumbar-sacral-iliac imbalance and malfunction (,the mother of scoliosis) and with the S.A.F.E.T.R.I.S. exercises to mobilize and correct that imbalance!!
 To recap ,"the precipitating factors "of this imbalance and malfunction of the lumbar-sacral-iliac joints, in other words "the mother cause " of scoliosis are :
 1) a true anatomical short leg, that's the TRUE SHORT LEG SCOLIOSIS according to my previous classification of scoliosis.
2) bad postural habits while sitting standing or walking, that's THE POSTURAL SCOLIOSIS, .according to my previous classification of scoliosis.

 3) direct or indirect trauma or strain to those joints, from falls, lifting, or twisting .and that includes the cause of idiopathic scoliosis in girls, THE BABYSITTING SCOLIOSIS.   And

<u>POST-TRAUMATIC SCOLIOSIS,</u>
<u>according to my previous classification</u>
<u>of scoliosis.</u>

<u>.</u>

<u>It is essential first to rule out a true</u>
<u>short leg as the cause of that imbalance,</u>
<u>"the mother cause" of scoliosis, because</u>
<u>as long as there is an anatomical short</u>
<u>leg that lumbar-sacral-Ilium imbalance</u>
<u>cannot be corrected.</u>

The other contributing factors of that
pelvic imbalance , 'the mother cause of
scoliosis," are bad postural habits and
strains and injuries to those lumbar-
sacral-iliac joints, should also be
eliminated.
By avoiding bad postural habits and
exercising daily with the right exercises
that pelvic imbalance will be corrected,
the progression of the abnormal spinal
curve will be stopped and even
eliminated<u>.</u>

<u>The purpose of the exercises is to restore the normal function of those joints and restore the balance to the base of the spine in order to prevent a small abnormal curve from becoming a huge curve requiring surgery with fusion and rods in the spine.</u>

When the 'mother cause of scoliosis" , the lumbar-sacral-Ilium joints imbalance return to its normal functioning state, the abnormal curve will reverse and go away the same way it was created PROVIDED that the functional scoliosis did not progressed to a structural scoliosis with real structural changes visible on the x-ray pictures.

 The Specific spinal exercises for the prevention and reduction of idiopathic scoliosis in short S.A.F.E.T.R.I.S.. are designed to mobilize, correct and return the normal function to the lumbar-sacral-iliac joints before any structural changes take place.

<u>The reason that many EXISTING conservative treatments and exercises are not very successful in treating the so called idiopathic scoliosis is simple. They do not remove the contributing factors of the mother   cause of scoliosis .</u> If you do not identify the contributing factor of "the mother cause" of scoliosis and remove it , no matter what treatments or exercises the patient has, the cause will keep causing the abnormal curve to return and even get worse. because the contributing factor is still   creating "the mother cause" of scoliosis!

It is time to recognize that the idiopathic scoliosis affecting kids and teenagers is a structural imbalance at the lumbar-sacral-pelvis joints **,(the mother cause of scoliosis)** caused by bad postural habits, falls, strains and injuries to those joints. The lumbar-sacral-pelvis joints are the foundation, the base of the spine and any injury , strain or malfunction to any of those joints will cause an abnormal spinal curve to form   with or without pain at the initial stage. That is why it is essential to recognize the contributing factors that cause the lumbar-sacral-iliac imbalance ",the mother cause of idiopathic scoliosis" and start the exercises early without any delay and wasting precious time.

It is time   to change the protocol for idiopathic scoliosis from the OBSERVATION period to an ACTION period to stop the progression of the abnormal spinal curve called scoliosis while the curve is still small, functional without any structural changes yet, and easier to reverse it. The one stitch in time (the small curve)to save nine (the severe abnormal curve) as the wise English proverb says.
The only way to stop the progression of scoliosis is to correct the cause of the abnormal curve, 'the mother of scoliosis', the lumbar-sacral-pelvic imbalance with the right exercises as soon as the initial diagnosis is made with the proper x-rays and eliminate any contributing factors. the true short leg, any bad postural habits, and the use of a small elastic support if necessary for protection and healing to take place.. .

-

10) IDIOPATHIC SCOLIOSIS.

FUNCTIONAL VERSUS STRUCTURAL IDIOPATHIC SCOLIOSIS

Idiopathic scoliosis of all ages with their fancy names, infantile, juvenile, adolescent, and adult idiopathic scoliosis, usually starts as a functional abnormal spinal curve at the lumbar-sacral- pelvic joints "the mother cause of scoliosis " and if not treated properly it will progress to a structural scoliosis with a severe abnormal spinal curve. The functional scoliosis with a small curve is easy to correct with spinal exercises and good postural habits.
If left untreated   and with bad postural habits , the functional scoliosis will progress to a structural scoliosis with structural and arthritic changes at the vertebral joints , thus making it more difficult to treat and life long suffering.

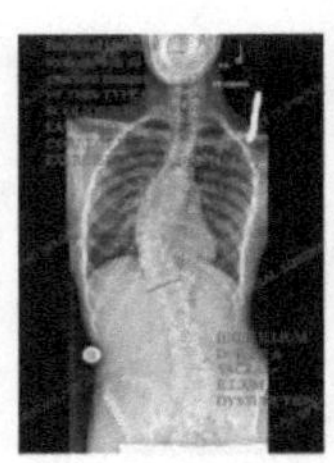 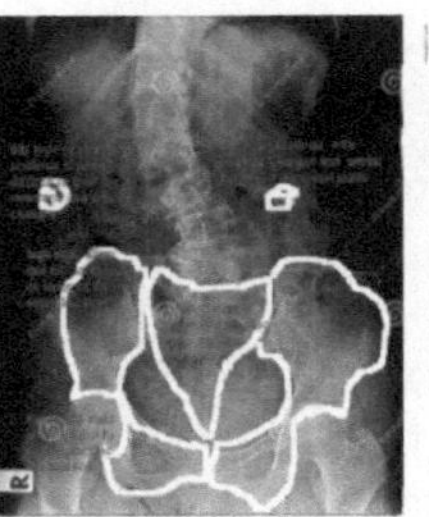

On the left is a functional idiopathic scoliosis with no structural changes yet. This type of scoliosis is easier to treat and reverse the abnormal curve with the S.A.F.E.T.R.I.S. EXERCISES.

The scoliosis on the right is a long standing structural scoliosis with arthritic changes at the vertebral joints. This structural scoliosis started out as a functional scoliosis with a small   curve, but because it was not treated properly it became a structural scoliosis with inflammation and arthritic changes. This type of scoliosis is very difficult to treat and almost impossible to reverse.

That is why it is very important to change the medical protocol for scoliosis treatment from the observation period to an action period to stop that small abnormal curve from becoming a big curve requiring spinal fusion and rods in the spine.

The difference between functional and structural scoliosis is the structural changes that take place at the vertebral joints.

With the functional idiopathic scoliosis when the patient bends forwards with   the Adam's test, the spine straightens out.

With the structural idiopathic scoliosis when the patient bends over the spine tries to straighten out but it cannot ,due to the structural changes to the spinal joints, inflammation and muscle spasm

 Both functional and structural idiopathic scoliosis started out as a small abnormal sideways functional CURVE and the longer it stays there, structural changes take place with   inflammation and arthritic changes. that is why it is very important to start the treatments with the spinal exercises early so it can prevent a small reversible curve from becoming a huge curve with vertebral joints changes and more difficult to treat and reverse.

 That is exactly the reason why the scoliosis treatment protocol should change from a wait and see approach, or the observation period, as it is called now , to an ACTION period to stop that small functional scoliosis from becoming a severe scoliosis needing   braces and spinal surgery with rods in the spine.

The Spinal Active Flexion Exercises to Reverse the Idiopathic scoliosis is the one stitch in time, (treatment of the small curve) to prevent nine (the huge abnormal curve). These exercises are specifically designed to treat the cause of the idiopathic scoliosis which is the lumbar-sacral-pelvis joints(THE MOTHER CAUSE OF SCOLIOSIS) and over time these joints to have a normal function, thus stopping the progression of the abnormal spinal curve.

The S,A,F,E,R,T,I,S, EXERCISES will be more effective making sure that there is not a true short leg and By eliminating the bad postural habits, practicing **good body mechanics** and exercising, so that the small functional idiopathic scoliosis will stop increasing and even reverse back to a normal straight spine.

What are body mechanics? Body mechanics is **the use of proper body movement to prevent and correct postural problems,   and enhance**

physical capabilities.

11)RESEARCH IS NEEDED

Research is needed to explore all the possibilities

how effectively to restore that lumbar- sacral-Ilium imbalance and joints malfunction" the mother cause of scoliosis" in the shortest possible time. **<u>Now we know that   this lumbar-sacral-iliac imbalance is the mother of the idiopathic functional and structural scoliosis</u>** and by restoring the balance and normal function to those joints will prevent a small abnormal spinal curve from becoming a huge abnormal curve   causing lifelong suffering. **<u>So the sooner the scientific community recognizes that this imbalance is "the mother of idiopathic scoliosis",, the sooner will conduct research on real people when they see that imbalance on the x-ray, which is ALWAYS there hiding in clear view for everyone to see it when they know what they are looking for .</u>**

Instead of ill -advising the patients to wait and see what happens in a years time , they will look for what really caused that lumbar-sacral-iliac imbalance, (the contributing factors). Was it a true anatomical short leg, or bad postural habits with strains and injuries to those joints. After ruling out a true short leg, they can advise the patients for good postural habits and exercising with S.A.F.E.T.R.I.S exercises to see how soon that imbalance will go away and normal function return to those joints.

Researchers are busy doing researches for years and they often come up with many theories as a causative factors for the idiopathic scoliosis. Theories born in a laboratory or in the figment of someone's vivid imagination are just theories and not a fact.

 It is time to forget the theories and look at the facts that are present on the x-rays of all scoliotic spines , THE MOTHER CAUSE OF SCOLIOSIS and the contributing factors to that lumbar-sacrum-iliac imbalance and malfunction.

The 'mother cause of idiopathic scoliosis" is clearly shown but hiding in clear view, on the x-ray pictures of every scoliotic spine, and that is a fact not a theory.

It is time to   question if the researchers   are on the right path doing the right researches? They explore the possibility of heredity, the DNA markers, etc, etc. I am just wondering why don't they look at the real patients with their   abnormal curves. If their feet are equal or not, if their postural habits are good or bad, if they had any falls injuries , strains in their spine?

And finally ,what do they have to say about the x-ray showings of every scoliotic spine with a clear imbalance at the lumbar-sacral-iliac joints   with a high Ilium on one side and the sacrum tilted on one side? Did they consider doing a research to find out the exact cause of that imbalance? Is it a short leg, bad postural habits, or strains and injury to that area? What happen when that imbalance and joint malfunction of the lumbar-sacral-iliac joints is restored? How soon that malfunction to those joints return to normal with the right exercises ? what happened to the abnormal curve when the base of the spine is leveled off? Of course it has to be reversed.

That is where all the spinal research should be done , the lumbar-sacral-pelvic joints., the base of the spine. Find out what caused that lumbar-sacra-pelvic joints imbalance, "THE MOTHER CAUSE OF SCOLIOSIS" and ways to restore the normal function of these joints to reverse the scoliotic curve, with the right spinal exercises.

 You do not even have to do a fancy research wasting huge amounts of money IN A STERILE LAB. As soon as an idiopathic scoliosis is diagnosed with X-rays showing no pathology present , and a clear lumbar-sacral-iliac imbalance is present," THE MOTHER OF SCOLIOSIS", advised the patient to avoid any bad postural positions and start the S.A.F.E.T.R.I.S. EXERCISES to correct any lumbar-sacrum-iliac dysfunction. When these joints are mobilized and have a normal anatomical function with a strong flexible spine the scoliosis will go away. The key is to start the exercises when the abnormal curve is still small and easy to correct. Above all the patient has to be informed of the cause of that abnormal curve and they have to have the motivation, the will and determination to do the exercises daily to stop the progression of the abnormal curve. NOBODY ELSE CAN DO THE EXERCISES FOR THEM! And unfortunately there is no magic pill to take and make the scoliosis go away.

 So instead of waiting to see how the spine will look in a year's time, they SHOULD exercise to stop the small curve from becoming a big curve.

THE MOTHER CAUSE OF IDIOPATHIC SCOLIOSIS

, is not an absurd theory created in a sterile laboratory but the real structural imbalance that caused the idiopathic scoliosis CLEARLY SHOWN on the x-rays of any idiopathic scoliosis, hiding in clear view for everyone to see it!

THE MOTHER CAUSE OF IDIOPATHIC SCOLIOSIS IS HIDING IN CLEAR VIEW ON EVERY X-RAY OF ANY SCOLIOTIC SPINE!!
x-ray pictures of idiopathic scoliosis clearly showing the lumbar-sacrum-iliac imbalance, the mother cause of every idiopathic scoliosis spine

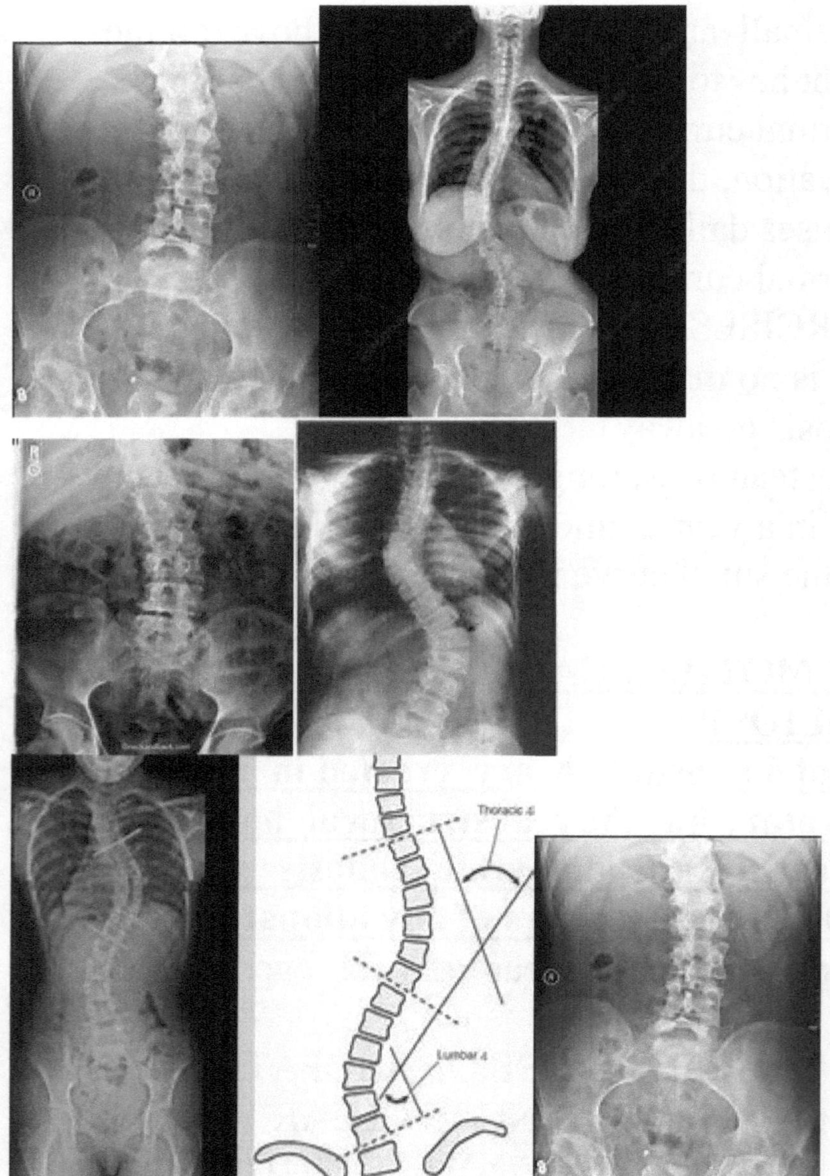

Thoracic 4
Lumbar 4

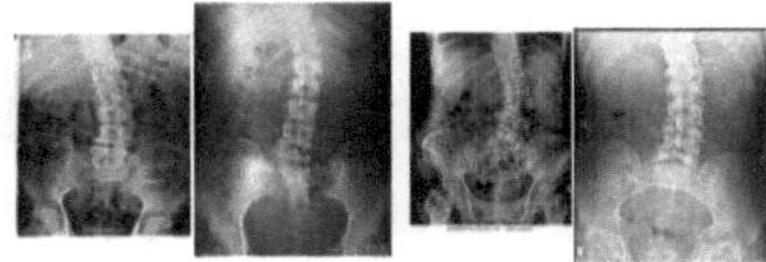

As a matter of fact one can create the idiopathic scoliosis by causing a structural imbalance to any of these three   lumbar-sacral-iliac joints, THE MOTHER OF SCOLIOSIS. But that would be cruel and inhumane!
 But if someone wants to volunteer to get a lumbar-sacral-iliac imbalance it can be done and a scoliosis will certainly start to form above that imbalance.

How can you create a lumbar- sacral-iliac imbalance ?

That is simple. Just create a functional short leg by removing the heel of one of your shoes and walk around with that created short leg and you will feel the imbalance of the lumbar-sacral-iliac joints right away. Before you know it a lumbar-sacral-iliac imbalance will be created and an abnormal spinal curve , the scoliosis will be born starting at that imbalance. To reverse it back to normal, just make sure that both shoes have equal heels otherwise that small functional scoliosis will keep growing. If left there for a long period of time that small functional scoliosis will progress to a structural scoliosis and a lifelong suffering.

Most of the time it is the sacroiliac joints that cause the whole structural imbalance by causing the sacrum to tilt at the side of the sacroiliac dysfunction . This can happen from a lifting accident, straining the sacroiliac joint forcing the Ilium on that side to go higher , creating a short leg on that side thus creating the perfect conditions for an abnormal spinal curve to start. The longer that imbalance remains the worse the abnormal spinal curve called idiopathic scoliosis will become and a secondary compensatory spinal curve in the thoracic spine will develop due to the righting reflex that the body tries to bring the center of gravity within its base, the sacrum and the two

feet.
What causes the imbalance to these key joints that cause the abnormal spinal curve called idiopathic scoliosis? Several factors. Bad postural habits while sitting standing or lying down. Bad body mechanics, Lifting accidents, girls lifting heavy babies, and that's the reason why more girls have scoliosis, accidental falls straining those joints creating a functional shot leg creating the perfect conditions for an abnormal curve to start. abnormal hugging, bear hugs, a child's tantrum, slips and falls , a true short leg due to a fracture or disease. All these are the factors that start the process for the lumbar-sacral- Ilium dysfunction and the creation of the abnormal spinal curve called idiopathic scoliosis. THE MOTHER CAUSE OF SCOLIOSIS.
Although the scientific community and the researchers and every one else for that matter, will never know when and what exactly caused that lumbar -sacral-iliac imbalance in every patient, because it is unique and different for each patient, THE IMPORTANT THING IS THAT WE KNOW FROM THE X-RAY PICTURES OF PEOPLE WITH SCOLIOSIS , that this lumbar -sacral- iliac imbalance CAUSES THE ABNORMAL SPINAL CURVE ABOVE . The important thing is that this imbalance and joints dysfunction is the causative factor for every

idiopathic scoliosis and it is present in every x-ray
picture of every scoliotic spine. When these joints
dysfunction and imbalance is corrected with the
spinal active flexion exercises to reduce the
idiopathic scoliosis and normalize the function of
these joints, the scoliosis will go away..
It is very important that as soon as the diagnosis of
the idiopathic scoliosis is made, to recognize how
bad that lumbar-sacral-pelvic imbalance is and
try to correct that imbalance as soon as possible
with the right exercises to stop the progression of
that abnormal curve.   Any delay in correcting that
imbalance the abnormal curve will keep getting
worse. So the prudent thing to do is not to delay
and waste valuable time wondering if it will
progress or improve.
The only way for that imbalance to correct itself is
only if the patient stopped the bad postural habits
by using proper body mechanics and started
exercising. Or if it was due to a strain or injury to
those joints, and that injury or strain healed after a
period of time by using a lumbar-sacral support for
protection and gave the nature a chance to heal
that strain..

This was also recognized by the famous
orthopedic surgeon Dr. John H .Moe who founded
the scoliosis research society and started his " DO
NOT DELAY CAMPAIGN.'   after one of his

patient died during spinal surgery.   The patient's old x-rays taken a few years earlier showing a mild scoliosis and because she did not get the proper treatment or support, her scoliosis progressed to a big curve requiring surgery and unfortunate she died during surgery making Dr. Moe furious and sad!

"Dr.. 'John H. Moe 1905-1988 a University of Minnesota orthopedic surgeon, who founded the Scoliosis Research Society in 1966 and he began a "do not delay" campaign for scoliosis, and he wrote   " procrastination was the most pernicious problem in idiopathic scoliosis and sad to see a child come with a severe curve requiring surgery with X-rays taken many years before showing a mild curve that could have been easily treated with a brace.46'Dangerous Curve" campaign "

It seems that after so many years of his famous campaign , the medical community still use the same archaic medical protocol of the "observation period " wasting precious time while the abnormal curve keeps growing causing serious health problems and sometimes requiring spinal fusion and rods in the patient's spine.

So it is prudent that as soon as the diagnosis of the idiopathic scoliosis is made, the patient should be instructed how to use proper body mechanics, avoid any bad postural habits, avoid lifting heavy

objects, or carrying any object on   one side of their
bodies. Advice them to use an elastic support or a
corset around their lumbar-sacral-pelvis joints for
protection from further injury, and start the right
exercises to normalize the function of those joints.
The spinal active flexion exercises to reduce
idiopathic scoliosis   in short S.A.F.E.R.T.I.S. are
designed to mobilize and restore the function of
the lumbar-sacral-pelvis joints and in the process
to stop the progression of the abnormal spinal curve
by making the spine stronger more flexible
without any abnormal curves.

12) DIAGNOSIS OF SCOLIOSIS

Anybody can see a crooked spine, but the proper diagnosis of scoliosis is made with x-rays and measuring the angle of the abnormal spinal curve with the COBB method. The angle measurements is to see the degree of the abnormal spinal curve. The greater the degree, the worse the scoliosis curvature is.
A scoliosis is defined as a lateral spinal curvature with a **Cobb** angle of 10° or more.

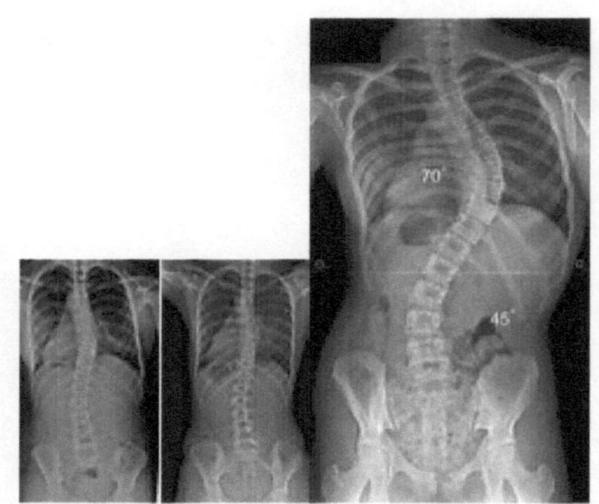

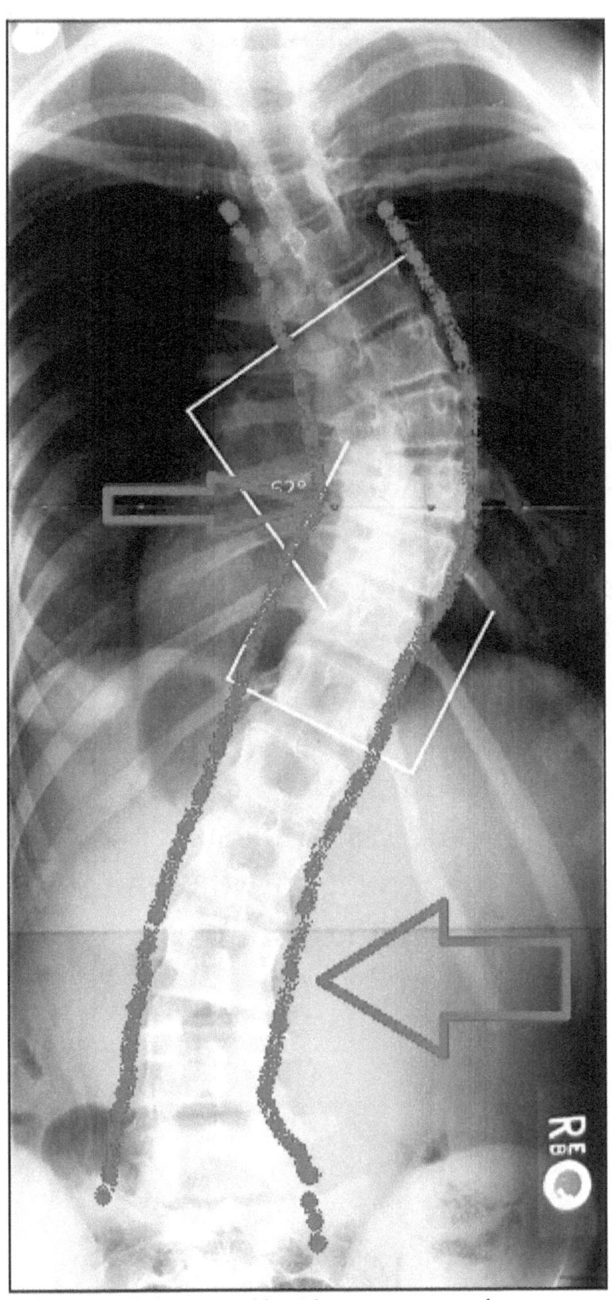

Idiopathic scoliosis x-ray pictures.
It is important to take x-rays of any scoliotic
spine to rule out any pathology, fractures or

anomalies of the spinal bones. If there is
pathology, fractures or anomalies in the bones then
the abnormal curve is due to that pathology or
fracture and requires immediate treatments by the
orthopedic specialist.

If there is no visible cause then it is the so called
idiopathic scoliosis and the patient is advised to
wait and see how that abnormal curve will develop
in a year or so by taking more x-rays.

However, since all the x-rays of the so called
idiopathic scoliosis show an imbalance of the
lumbar-sacral-iliac joints, which in my opinion
that is **the mother cause of every idiopathic
scoliosis**, I think it is about time to pay more
attention to that imbalance and stop calling the
idiopathic scoliosis ,   IDIOPATHIC.

We call the so called idiopathic scoliosis according
to the causative factors that precipitate the lumbar-
sacral-iliac imbalance creating the scoliosis,
according to my classification below.

13) NEW CLASSIFICATION OF IDIOPATHIC SCOLIOSIS

In my book , " SCOLIOSIS:: A FRESH LOOK AT WHAT CAUSES THE IDIOPATHIC FUNCTIONAL SCOLIOSIS AND HOME EXERCISES TO STOP THE PROGRESSION OF THE CURVE AND EVEN REVERSE IT BACK TO NORMAL "   I classified the idiopathic scoliosis according to the causative factors contributing to the lumbar-sacral-iliac imbalance and joint malfunctions that causes the creation of the abnormal spinal curve called scoliosis.

1)**<u>POSITIONAL INFANTILE SCOLIOSIS</u>** (from the old infantile idiopathic scoliosis which is caused when the mother or care giver hold the babies on one side of their body or they always place the babies in one side when they sleep.) that prolong position in one side creates scoliosis and plagiocephaly.

2)BAD HABITS POSTURAL JUVENILE AND ADOLESCENT SCOLIOSIS OR <u>**JUST**</u>

<u>**POSTURAL JUVENILE AND ADOLESCENT SCOLIOSIS**</u> (from the old idiopathic adolescent scoliosis ,which is caused by bad postural habits in their daily lives. The bad postural habits are contributing factors of the mother cause of scoliosis.

 3)BABYSITTING JUVENILE AND ADOLESCENT SCOLIOSIS (from the old juvenile and adolescent idiopathic scoliosis that affect more girls than boys and the cause is babysitting or lifting and playing with heavy babies, which causes strain and injuries to the lumbar-sacral iliac joints, the mother of scoliosis)

 4)TRAUMATIC COMPENSATORY JUVENILE AND ADOLESCENT SCOLIOSIS (from the old idiopathic juvenile and adolescent scoliosis)this type of scoliosis is due to untreated strains, sprains, or other injuries to the low back and pelvic joints. or by just kids being kids fooling around or playing practical jokes or even bending down to pick their ball and can get a low back strain .) this creates an imbalance at lumbar-sacral-iliac joints and malfunction of these joints, creating the perfect conditions for the abnormal spinal curve to develop. Again the strains and injuries are contributing factors that create "the mother cause of scoliosis"

 5) TRUE SHORT LEG COMPENSATORY
JUVENILE AND   ADOLESCENT SCOLIOSIS (
From the old idiopathic juvenile adolescent
scoliosis, when there is a true short leg .) AGAIN
the true short leg is contributing to the creation of"
the mother cause of scoliosis."

These are the new classification of the idiopathic
scoliosis according to the contributing factors that
are responsible for the lumbar-sacral-iliac
imbalance 'THE MOTHER CAUSE OF
SCOLIOSIS" that cause scoliosis.

14) EXISTING TREATMENTS FOR SCOLIOSIS

According to the present medical protocol ,
treatments for the idiopathic scoliosis, is:
  a) observation which is a waste of precious time,
 b) bracing when the abnormal curve gets worse
and
 c) surgery with spinal fusion and rods in the spine.

I think the worst part of the protocol is the
observation period   with the waste of precious time
by doing nothing for the small treatable curve and
watch that small curve getting worse requiring
braces and even   surgery as time goes by. Braces
can be somewhat effective if the causative factors
are bad postural habits and with the braces the
patients are forced to correct their bad postural
habits. Braces can also be very useful if the
contributing factors are sprains or strains .the
braces provide support of those joints and enables
healing to take place.
Surgery with spinal fusion and rods in the spine
are necessary when the abnormal curve is severe
and causes respiratory or other difficulties.

d)The existing conservative treatments for the
idiopathic scoliosis are physiotherapy , exercises,

traction , manipulation and other methods.
Some of the conservative treatments are good,
some of them are so- so and some of them are not
good and a waste of time and money.
 However none of the conservative treatments are
taking into consideration the cause of the
abnormal spinal curve. They treat the abnormal
curve as idiopathic scoliosis , meaning that they do
not know what is causing that crooked spine and
if they do not know the cause , they cannot treat it
properly. In other words the treatments are
experimental and some times they can be effective
and other times not effective.
The reason that many conservative treatments are
not effective, is that they do not recognize the '''the
mother cause of scoliosis' the lumbar-sacrum-iliac
imbalance and the contributing factors that cause
that imbalance. They fail to recognize and remove
the contributing factors.
In order to treat any condition effectively , first
you have to identify the cause of that condition and
remove that   cause so that the treatments are
effective. Otherwise no matter what you do if the
causative factors are still there they will continue
to make the abnormal curve worse. For example if
the abnormal curve of scoliosis is caused by an
anatomical short leg, no matter what treatments or
exercises that patient does, it will not correct that
curve, because the true shot leg will keep causing

lumbar-sacral-iliac imbalance forcing the spine into a scoliotic curve. The proper way to treat that scoliosis effectively is to correct the length of the short leg   first ,and then do the proper exercises or treatments .

That is why I gave the idiopathic scoliosis new names with the plausible cause. In order to have good results and correct that abnormal curve is to remove the cause, the contributing factors that precipitate the lumbar-sacral-iliac imbalance, the mother cause of scoliosis.

Once the contributing factor is removed and eliminated , it is time to start the S.A.F.E.T,R,.I.S.. exercises.

I designed these exercises based on the Adam's forward bend observation, in which the functional scoliosis is straighten out and the structural scoliosis tries to straighten out. The exercises are designed to put all the spinal joints through their normal range of motion and with repetition to strengthen the muscles and ligaments of those joints and in the process to make the spine stronger more flexible without any abnormal curves. The exercises are spinal stretches, easy to do and there is no need for any equipment. You can do them in the privacy of your own home on a mat or even in your own bed.

As I mention above, these exercise will be more effective when the abnormal curve is still small

and easier to stop the progression of scoliosis and
even reverse it back to normal .   But these
exercises will help increase the mobility and
flexibly of any scoliotic spine , so it is worth
trying these exercises. You also have to eliminate
any bad postural habits , use an elastic support to
lumbar-sacral-iliac joints for support and
promoting   healing if there is any strain there.
The purpose of the spinal active flexion exercises
is to reduce idiopathic scoliosis, in short
S.AF..F.T.R.I.S. is to correct the lumbar -sacral-
iliac imbalance and malfunction of those joints.
ELIMINATING BAD POSTURAL HABITS IS
ESSENTIAL FOR THE EXERCISES TO BE
EFFECTIVE.

 Below are the   exercises with pictures.

15) THE   SPINAL ACTIVE FLEXION
EXERCISES TO REDUCE IDIOPATHIC
SCOLIOSIS in short (S.A.F.E.T.R.I.S.)

In my previous books I called these exercises
Spinal Active Flexion Exercises in short S,A.F.E.

but that did not explain what these exercises are
for , so I had to add to that acronym to indicate
that they were for the reduction of idiopathic
scoliosis, S.A.F.E.T.R.I.S. spinal active flexion
exercises to reduce idiopathic scoliosis.
These exercises are designed to stretch, mobilize
and put all the spinal joints from the head to the
coccyx, including the lumbar-sacral- pelvic joints
, and rib joints through their normal range of
motion. By exercising at least twice daily, all the
joints will be mobilized, stretched , corrected ,
retain   their normal range of motion and in the
process to make the spine stronger and more
flexible without any abnormal curves.
The key for a healthy spine without any abnormal
curves is the right spinal exercises.
There are many spinal exercises out there but some
of them cause more harm than good to the spine,
especially the ones that go contrary to the normal
range of the spinal joints, like the rotation with
extension which make any crooked spine worse.

Basic precaution and instructions.

In order to reduce the abnormal spinal curve
faster you have to eliminate your old bad postural
habits. Avoid slouching when you sit at home ,

school or work. For the girls with their mother
instinct, they should avoid lifting or holding babies
which is the major cause why girls have scoliosis
more often than   the boys. The so called
babysitting   scoliosis , which I described in my
book: GIRLS' SCOLIOSIS.

**N.B. You do these exercises on an empty
stomach and never after a meal or a big drink.
YOU ALWAYS TAKE IT EASY AND NEVER
STRAIN YOURSELF.**

**If any exercise causes pain , skip it and do
another exercise until you are stronger and
more flexible.**

**If you have low back pain it is advisable to use
an elastic support or corset during the day,
especially in the beginning when you start
exercising, but not for long period times .
Prolong use of braces causes muscle weakness
and stiffness.**

**Avoid any spinal extension exercises. With the
scoliosis the bones of the spine are crowded ,
twisted and jammed and any extension
exercises aggravates the crowding bones making
the scoliosis worse!!**

These exercises are easy to do in the privacy of your home even in your own bed, or a mat on the floor of your room.

<u>For the kids with idiopathic scoliosis it is advisable to be supervised by their Parents or a therapist in the beginning.</u>

<u>It is also advisable to get your doctor advice before starting any strenuous exercises, to make sure that there are no contraindications to exercise.</u>

For all the kids and especially girls they should avoid lifting or holding other kids or anything else for that matter.
<u>Lifting heavy kids is the number one cause of the girls' scoliosis.</u>

And finally Make sure you do not wear any tight clothing while you exercise.
Comfortable gym clothes of well fitted pajamas are perfect .
 sleeping clothes: a light loose pair of pants and a matching loose-fitting shirt or top for wearing in bed or for lounging are ok.
You have to be comfortable while you exercises.

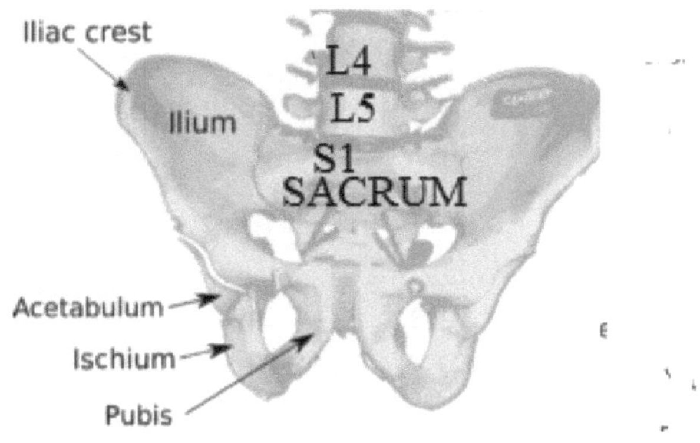

Correcting the mother cause of scoliosis, the lumbar-sacral-iliac imbalance and malfunction, with the spinal active flexion exercises to reduce idiopathic scoliosis, in short S.A.F.E.R.T.I.S.

**16) DESCRIPTIONS OF THE   HOME
S.A.F.ET.R.I.S) EXERCISES .**

 **HERE ARE THE   HOME EXERCISES WHICH I
DESIGNED AND I CALL S.A.F.ET.R.I.S. (SPINAL
ACTIVE FLEXION EXERCISES TO REDUCE
IDIOPATHIC SCOLIOSIS)**

EXERCISE ONE.

Make sure you do not wear any tight clothing
while you exercise.
Comfortable gym clothes of well fitted pajamas.
 sleeping clothes: a light loose pair of pants and a
matching loose-fitting shirt or top for wearing in
bed or for lounging are ok.
You have to be comfortable while you exercises.

Lie face up on a mat or a mattress ,
Interlock your fingers and place them under your head.

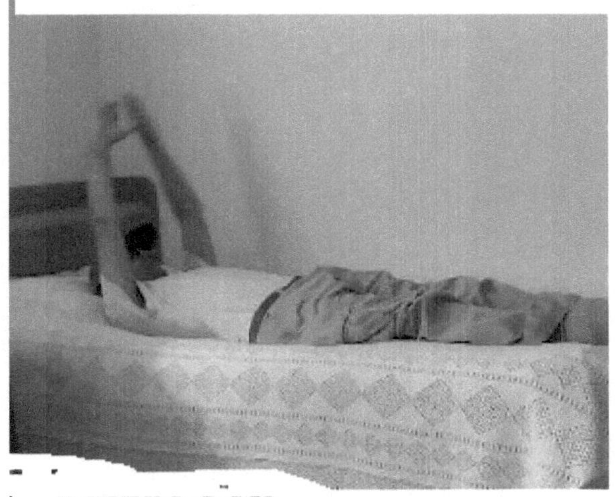

Take a deep breath in expanding your chest as much as possible. times.

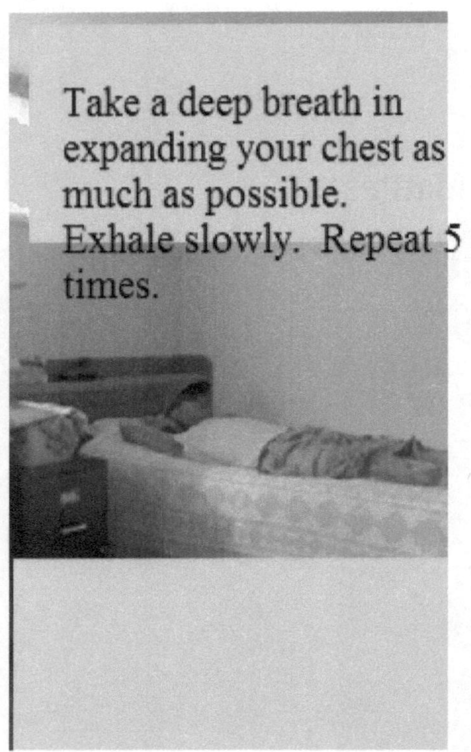

This exercise is good for expanding your chest cavity stretching your ribs and your shoulder blades.. it will exercise and strengthen the chest muscles and will restore normal range of motion to the ribs reducing any rib hump

Exercise two
Lying face up with your hands
interlocked under your head

Then bring your bent elbows towards your nose as
far as you can

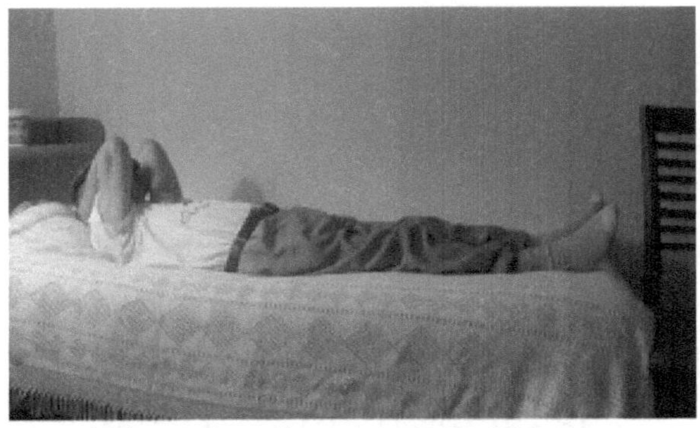

And then back towards the mattress pressing on the
mattress.

lying face up,
interlock fingers
and place them
under your head

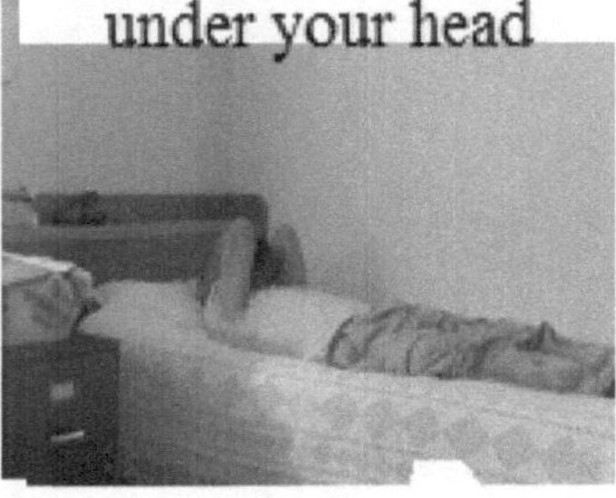

bring your elbows
towards your face ,
then back pressing on
the mattress

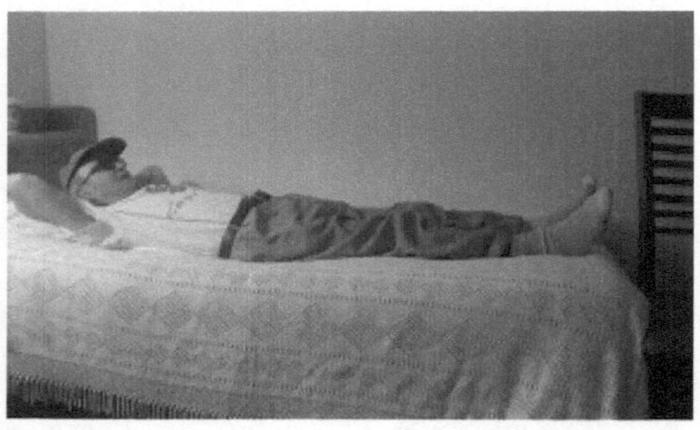

Repeat this motion of your elbows towards your
nose and back to pressing on the mattress 10-20
times.
Do not overdo it but keep increasing the
repetitions as you get stronger.
These exercises are the best for strengthening your
upper chest and shoulder muscles and mobilizing

your upper thoracic and cervical spine.

Rest   by taking deep breaths expanding your
chest as much as possible and exhaling slowly.

EXERCISE THREE

From the same position, face up, hands interlocked
behind the head
Bend your right knee and let it down   on the
mattress
  and raise your head towards the chest   as far as
you can without straining yourself.
  Repeat 5 times and keep increasing them as you

get stronger. Never over do it .

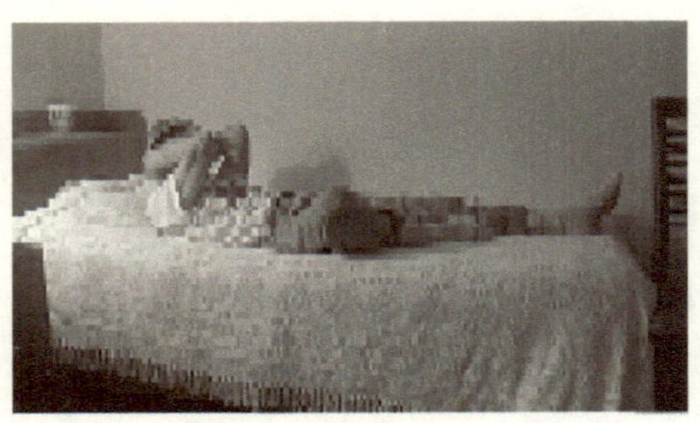

Repeat the same exercise with your left knee
  Bend your left knee ,
Let it down on you left side
and raise the head towards your chest five times

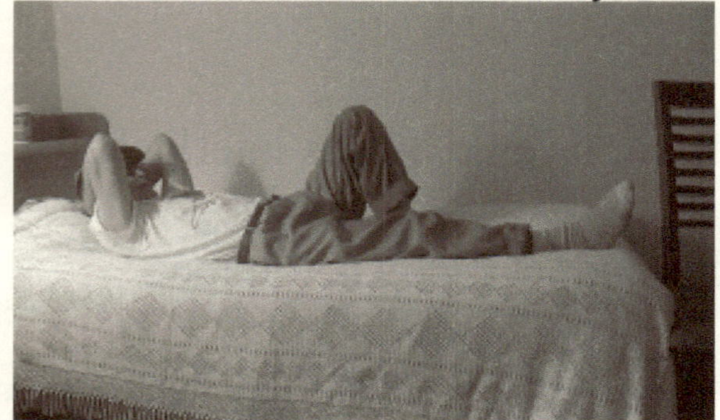

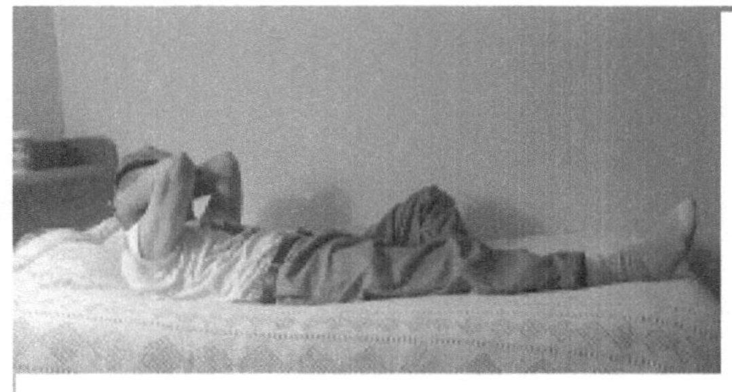

Repeat this exercise 5 times and as you get stronger and more flexible you increase the repetitions.

N.B. This is not a sit up exercise and do not try to sit up, you just raise your head towards your chest to stretch your spine as much as possible without straining yourself .

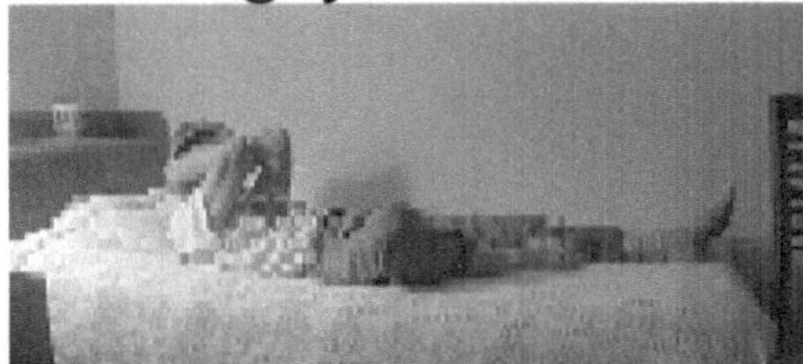

lying face up, bend
right knee and let it
down on right side on
mat

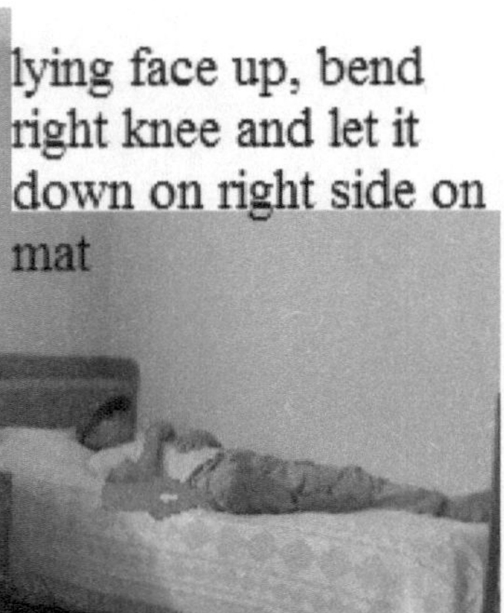

push your right knee
towards your other foot

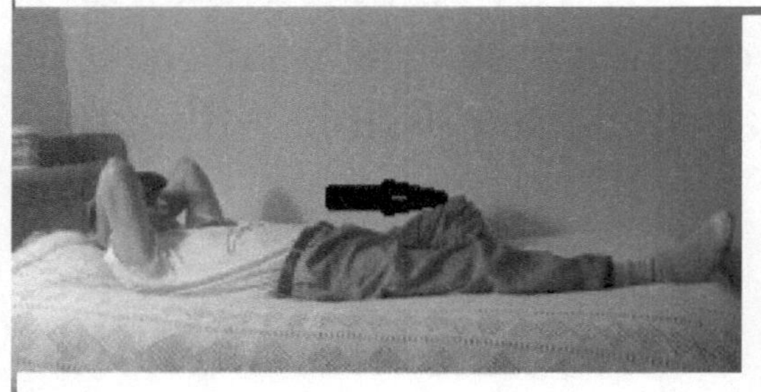

Knee to the side and push the knee down towards
the other foot

These exercise are very good at stretching and correcting any misalignments normalizing the function of the lumbar-sacrum-iliac joints.

Rest   by taking   5 deep breaths in by expanding your chest as much as possible and exhaling slowly.

Exercise four

The moving bridge.

Lying down face up with your   interlocked hand
fingers under your head.
 Bend your knees and raise your low back towards
the ceiling and down to the mattress , up and down
10-20 times. Go easy and never strain yourself
and as you get stronger increase the repetitions.

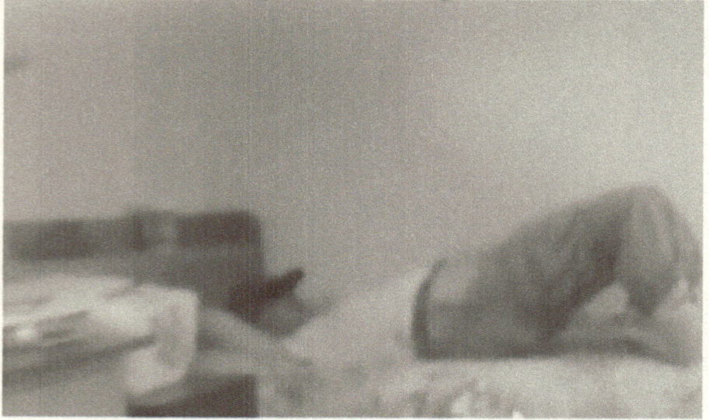

This exercise strengthens your abdominal , spinal
and leg muscles and mobilizes the hip and
sacroiliac joints.

Rest   by taking 5 deep breaths in expanding
your chest as much as possible and exhaling
slowly.

Exercise five

Bend your right knee and bring it   towards your
chest and raise your head towards your knee.
Repeat this   exercise 5 times

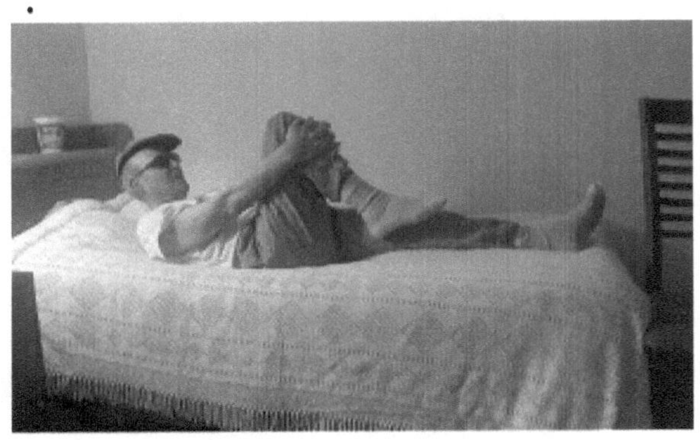

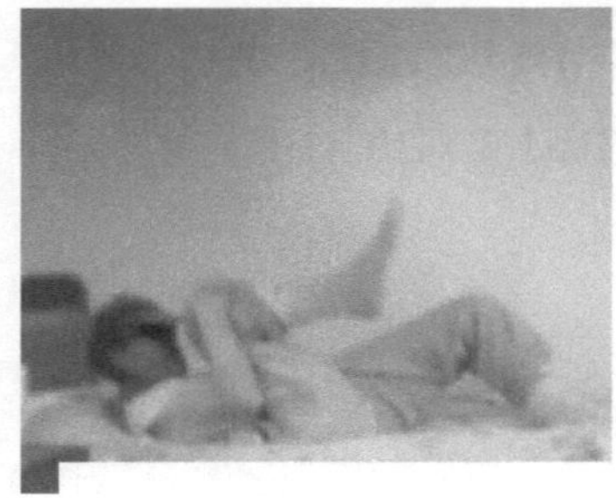

Repeat the same exercise with your left knee

Repeat the same exercise with your left knee

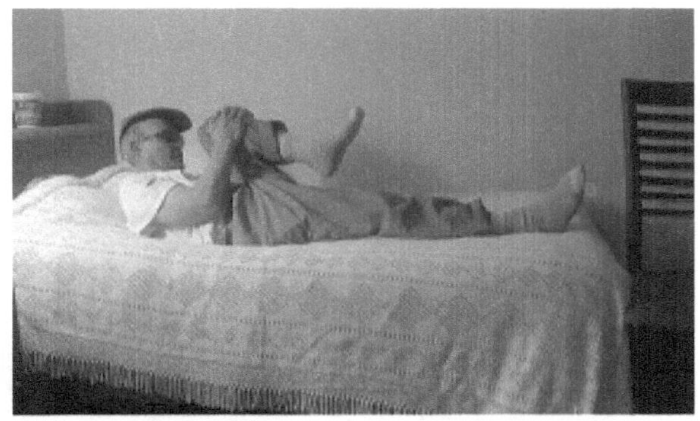

These exercises are very good to reduce any misalignments to the sacrum -iliac joints and sacrum lumbar vertebrae..   Also good for the abdominal muscles and   good for all spinal joints stretch from the sacrum to the upper cervical vertebrae.

"This exercise makes positive changes in the joints, along with increasing the blood supply promoting healing by supplying necessary nutrients into the area for healing."

Exercise six

Knees to chest exercises with   raising your head towards your knees.
Bend your knees and bring them to your chest as close as possible , without straining yourself
And raise your head towards your knees
Hold that position to the count of three
Repeat this exercise 5 times without straining yourself and as you get stronger you increase the repetitions by 1-2 every few days

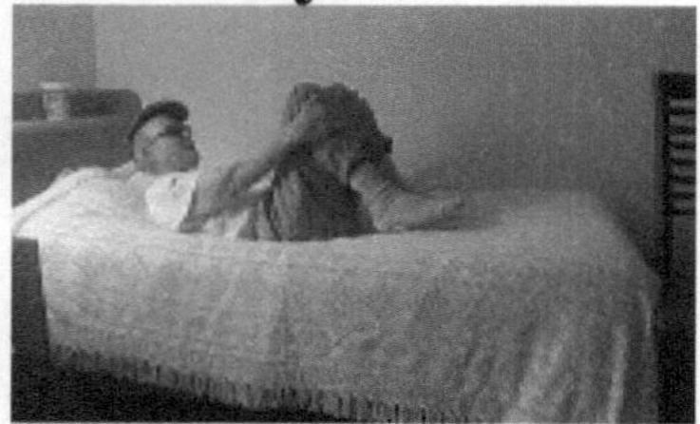

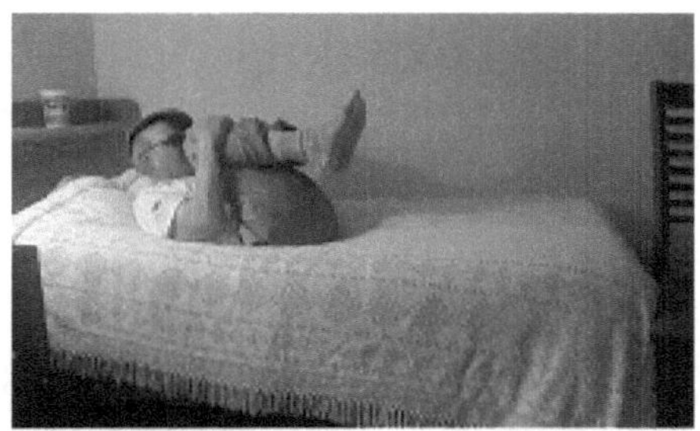

Go easy on yourself and do not over do it.

This exercise is good at mobilizing all the joints of your spine, hips and pelvis and increases the flexibility of the spine and   pelvis. It is a very good spinal stretch that increases the flexibility of the spine, increases the blood supply and promotes healing .

THIS IS A VERY IMPORTANT EXERCISE, AND THIS IS THE MAXIMUM (FLEXION) BEND FORWARD THAT MIMICS THE ADAMS TEST STRETCHING THE SPINE TO ITS MAXIMUM WITHOUT GRAVITY.

This exercise stretches the whole spine promoting good range of motion correcting any misalignments . It also straightens the spine , and over time it will reduce the abnormal spinal curve called idiopathic scoliosis.
Rest   by taking 5 deep breaths in expanding

your chest as much as possible and exhaling
slowly.

 If there is any pain during the exercises, stop and
rest, and do the exercises that are easy for you and
pain free first and then gradually as you get
stronger and more flexible you do the more
difficult exercises.

Exercise seven

KNEES TO CHEST ROCKING EXERCISE

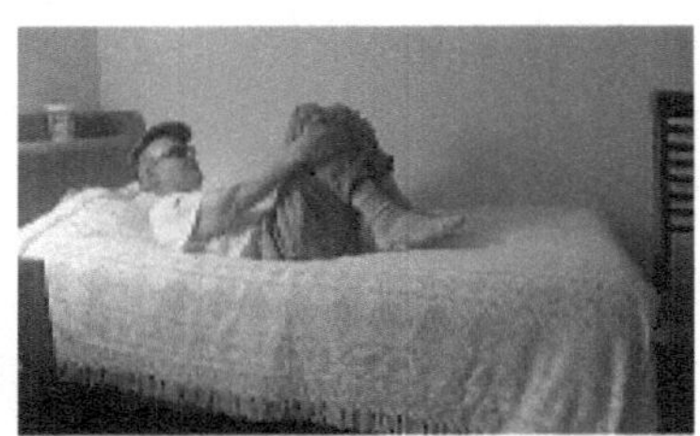

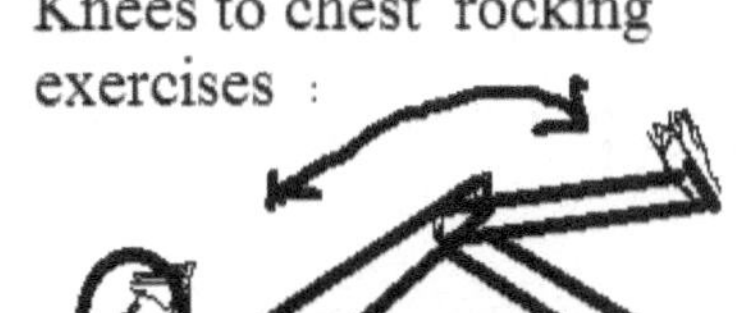

this is the most
important exercise
to increase the
flexibility of your
spine.

grab your right knee with your right
hand and your left knee with your left
hand and bring your knees to your
chest and with a rocking motion rock
your pelvis back and forth

**THIS EXERCISE MOBILIZES ALL JOINTS OF
THE SPINE, HIP
AND PELVIS JOINTS AND CHEST AND**

SHOULDER JOINTS

Bring your bent knees towards your chest
Grab your right knee with your right hand
And your left knee with your left hand

While holding your knees with your hands
about 6- 12 inches apart

WITH A ROCKING MOVE

Rock your pelvis back and forth
by bringing your knees to your chest
And back without your feet touching the mat

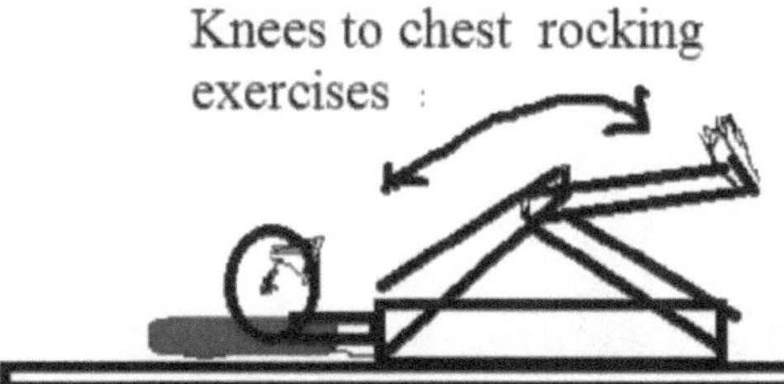

Knees to chest rocking exercises : this is the most important exercise to increase the flexibility of your spine.

grab your right knee with your right hand and your left knee with your left hand and bring your knees to your chest and with a rocking motion rock your pelvis back and forth

REPEAT THIS EXERCISE 10-20 TIMES WITHOUT STRAINING YOUR SELF And increase the repetition every week by 5 until you reach 100 or more, depending on your physical condition and stamina. Remember never to overdo it or strain yourself.

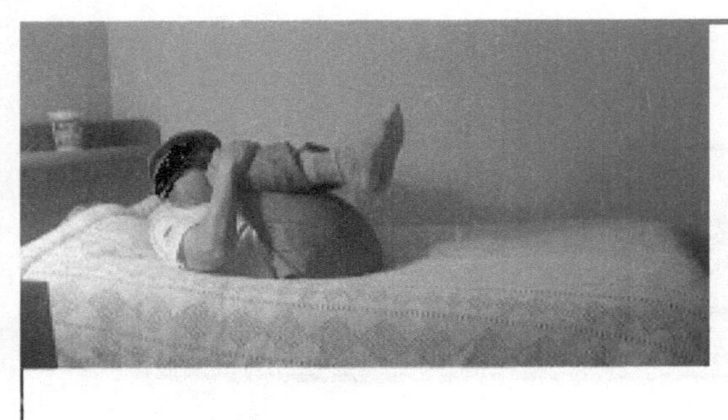

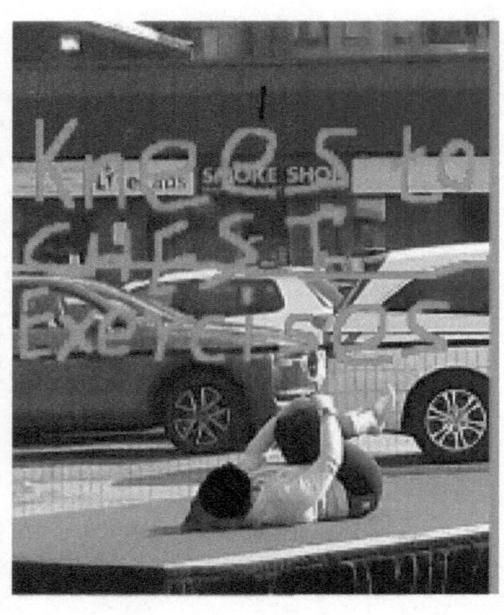

**This exercise is very good at mobilizing all the joints of your
spine, hips and pelvis, chest and shoulders.**

**Increases the flexibility of the spine and   pelvis
and strengthens the muscles of the spine. This
exercise will correct any misalignments at the
sacrum-lumbar - pelvis area and make those
joints stronger.**
**This exercise promotes healing and regeneration
on any damaged** intervertebral disk disease by
increasing the blood supply to the area. It is also
good for the structural idiopathic scoliosis to
increase the range of motion of the spinal joints,
reduce muscle spasm and promote healing to any
damage of the inter-vertebral discs but you have to
go easy and it will take a long time to notice the
improvements. But still it is worth trying them and
exercising daily.

**Go easy on yourself and do not over do it, with
time as you get stronger and more flexible you
will be able to do more.**
**As your spine is getting stronger and more
flexible   the Cobb angle will be getting smaller
and your spine straighter .**

N.B. this knees to chest exercise should be done by
everyone from age one to   old age to maintain
the strength and flexibility of the spine.

Exercise 8

SACROILIAC joints SPINAL STRETCH

Lying face up , bend your right knee and let it down on the mat,
Your right foot is touching your left thigh.
Push your right knee downwards in the direction of your left foot,
Repeat 3-5 times on each knee

lying face up, bend
right knee and let it
down on right side on
mat

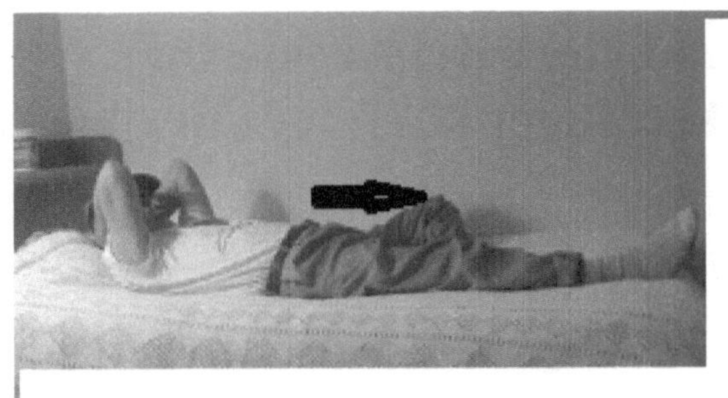

push your right knee
towards your other foot

Repeat this exercise 5 times

Repeat the same exercise on left side

This exercise is   stretching , mobilizing and correcting the sacroiliac, and sacrum-L5 joints

Exercise nine

SPINAL STRETCH raising the head to chest with the hands behind the head

N.B. this is not a sit up exercise. Do not try to sit up.

Lying face up, hands behind the head,
Bring your elbows towards your face
And raise your head towards your chest without straining yourself and then lower you head gently to the mattress.
Repeat it 3-5 times and you can increase the repetitions as you get stronger and more flexible

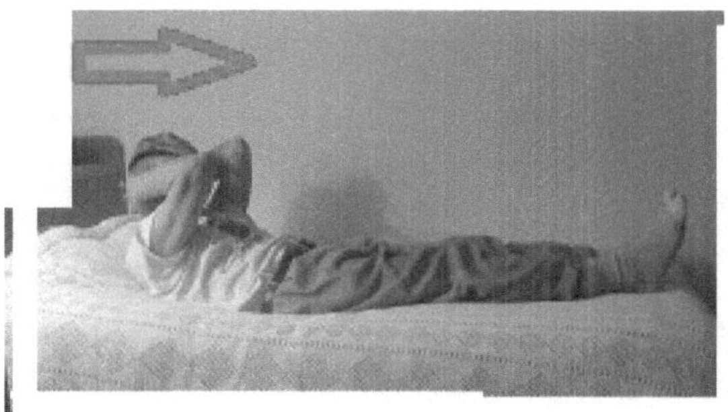

lying face up,hands behind the head
bring elbows towards the face
and raise your head towards your
chest and then gently down

**This exercise stretches and mobilizes the spinal joints from the pelvis to the head.
Go easy and do not overdo it but keep increasing the number of repetitions as you get stronger and more flexible.**

Exercise   ten

You finish with the same exercise as the number one exercise

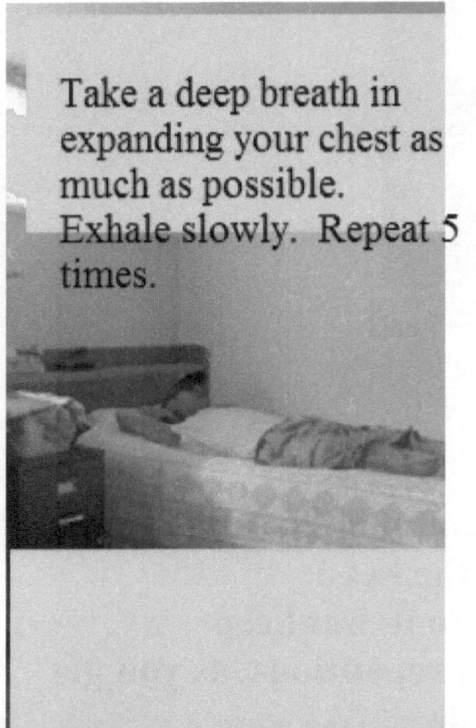

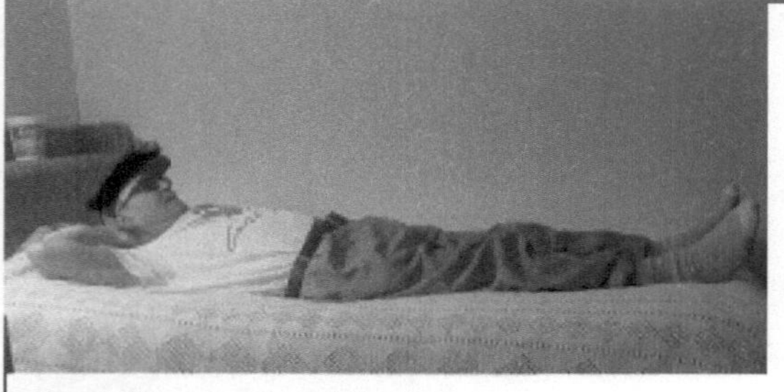

lying face up with your
handsbehindyour head
take a deep breath in expanding your
chest as much as possible
and then exhaling slowly
repeat X 5 times

This exercise is good for expanding your chest
cavity stretching your ribs and your shoulder
blades.. it will exercise, and strengthen the chest

muscles . It will also mobilize and restore the normal range of motion to the ribs reducing any rib hump.

N.B. You do these exercises on an empty stomach and never after a meal, or   a big drink.

YOU ALWAYS TAKE IT EASY AND NEVER STRAIN YOURSELF .

If some exercise causes pain , skip it and do another exercise until you are stronger and more flexible.

**N.B. DO THESE EXERCISES 2- 3 TIMES A DAY
 UNLESS YOU ARE SICK OR HAVE FEVER IN WHICH CASE YOU DO NOT DO ANY EXERCISES**

These are the exercises that have the potential to stop the progression of the abnormal spinal curves and even reverse the spine back to normal. These exercises put all the spinal joins

within their normal range of motion and strengthen the ligaments and all the spinal muscles, thus making the spine stronger and more flexible.

 N.B. FOR BETTER RESULTS, REMEMBER TO STOP ANY BAD POSTURAL HABITS YOU AND REPLACE THEM WITH GOOD POSTURAL HABITS BY AVOIDING SLOUCHING POSITIONS WHEN YOU SIT, STAND OR WALKING.

17)   FOR BETTER RESULTS KEEP A DAILY DIARY.

When you start doing the s.a.f.e.t.r.i.s. spinal exercises keep a daily diary to check your progress   and the most important thing is to keep focus , positive and avoid slouching positions, heavy lifting , especially heavy babies.

Take a picture of your spine just before starting

the exercises and re-take pictures of your spine every week to see the progress you are making.

You should see some improvements in your spine in 4-6 weeks and as the time goes by, your spine will be stronger and more flexible. Any abnormal curves will start to improve and reduced.

Everyday write down exactly how you do the exercises, how many times you do each exercise and how you feel during and after the exercises.

Remember   never to strain yourself or overdo it, and as you get stronger and more flexible increase the repetitions of each exercise.

 THE DAILY DIARY   WILL MOTIVATE AND ENCOURAGE YOU WHEN YOU START SEEING IMPROVEMENTS IN YOUR SCOLIOSIS.

As time goes by and you feel stronger increase the repetitions
And the time you do them. More repetitions means stronger muscles and   more flexible spine.

The most important thing is that you do these exercises to get better , healthier, more

flexibility and above all to stop the progression
of any abnormal curves and reduce   the angle
of your scoliosis.
Even when your spine feels better and your
scoliosis is reduced, keep doing these exercises
at least once a day to keep your spine strong,
healthy and flexible.

Get into the habit to do them every morning
when you get up before you have any breakfast.

Always remember that exercises and good
nutrition is the mother of good health, good
posture and longevity with good quality of life.

18) EXPECTED RESULTS WITH THE S.A.F.E.T.R.I.S.

The S.A.F.E.T.R.I.S. .   exercises are designed to give flexibility and strength to the spine as long as you do them daily.

To have good results you have to <u>change your old habits of bad posture at home, at school and avoid slouching everywhere else</u>.

If you do the exercises and keep doing what you have been doing that started the scoliosis, do not expect much, because you did not remove the CAUSE, 'the bad postural habits" that started the scoliosis in the first place.

You might see some improvement but not as much as   when you removed the cause, the bad posture habits and lifting of heavy objects including heavy babies or school bags.

if you do the exercises daily three times a day and you removed the cause of the scoliosis, and if you are a girl you should stop lifting and carrying babies around **. With these exercises along with some swimming exercises and monkey bar stretching exercises you should get good results in 2-3 months . These exercises should stop the progression of the abnormal curve called scoliosis and the Cobb angle of your scoliosis should start to get smaller and smaller with time.**

<u>**OF COURSE** your improvement will depend</u>

<u>on the effort you put into the exercises and your
avoidance of what causes the scoliosis, such as
lifting heavy objects, slouching, when you sit   at
home, in class and walking.</u>

Even when you see some improvement you
should keep doing the exercises daily for ever . if
you want to have a strong ,healthy, flexible
spine, along with all the other health benefits
that come with a healthy spine, like good health,
good looks and good posture.
The exercises will be taking you about 15
minutes times 3 a total of 45 minutes a day and
the health benefits are enormous . Besides you
do not waste time going to a gym and you need
no equipment to do the exercises.
<u> Of course you will be doing these exercises on an
empty stomach and you should not exercise when
you are sick with fever , infections or have severe
pain.</u>

 I am not a fun or believer of "NO PAIN NO
GAIN." slogan.
 When there is pain, it is a warning from your
body to stop and you should always listen to
your body. DO the exercises that do not cause
any pain and gradually do more. Let your body
guide you what exercises are suitable for you!

19) HERE ARE SOME MORE GOOD EXERCISES FOR THE PREVENTION AND CORRECTION OF SCOLIOSIS

More good exercises that have the potential to prevent and help you have a strong healthy and flexible spine without any abnormal curves.

Here are some of the best exercises to prevent and treat   scoliosis.

1)Swimming: swimming is an excellent exercise for preventing scoliosis and if you can swim , swim every time you have the chance. Fishes swim all the time and they never get scoliosis.

2)Monkey bar exercises are very good for stretching exercises of the spine. Spinal stretch or pull up exercises. The monkeys do these exercises all the time and they do not have any

scoliosis.

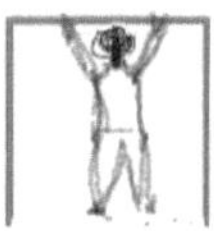

3)Modified Adam's   forward bending test which I described in detailed in my book : how to prevent and treat scoliosis.
The modified Adam's forward bending test exercise is done by: START WITH THE STANDING POSITION
 Your feet are placed 12 inches apart
Bend forwards from the waist without bending your knees
And touch your left foot   with your right fingers
While your left hand is at the back of your low back

Come up to straight position

 And then bend forwards from your waist and touch your right foot with the fingers of your left hand while your right hand is placed at your low back

N.B. if you have a noticeable rib hump on your right side,
Then do twice as many bends forwards with your right hand
To your left foot, and vice versa.

This is done because when you bend forwards and bring your right hand(the same side of your rib hump) to your left foot,   the bending forwards stretches and brings forwards the rib hump and corrects your rib cage
And with time it should bring it back to its normal position.

That is why you do the forwards bends twice as much on the side of the rib hump.

START WITH THE STANDING POSITION BUT
YOUR FEET ARE PLACED 12-18 INCHES APART
BEND FORWARDS AND TOUCH YOUR LEFT
FOOT WITH YOUR RIGHT HAND FINGERS
WHILE YOUR LEFT HAND RESTS ON THE BACK
OF YOUR LOW BACK

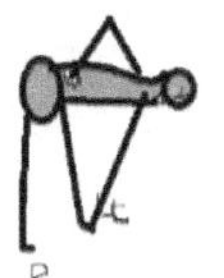

START WITH THE STANDING POSITION BUT
YOUR FEET ARE PLACED 12-18 INCHES APART
BEND FORWARDS AND TOUCH YOUR LEFT
FOOT WITH YOUR RIGHT HAND FINGERS
WHILE YOUR LEFT HAND RESTS ON THE BACK
OF YOUR LOW BACK

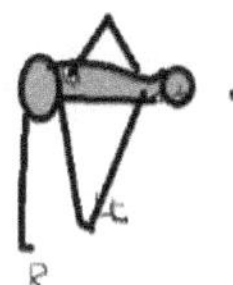

20) EXERCISES TO AVOID

 Good exercises will make your spine strong,
healthy, flexible and will safeguard your spine from
any injury.

Bad exercises will   have the potential to cause
injury to the spine and even cause chronic
debilitating diseases and scoliosis.

Avoid all extension and twisting exercises. They
can cause injuries to the spine and the beginning of
scoliosis at any age,

Avoid lifting exercises   unless you have a low
back support and you bend your knees. Watch how
the weight lifters train   and exercise with weights.
 Stop any exercise that cause pain. Pain is a
warning that whatever you do is not good for the
body.
 Avoid any warm up stretches that require bending
and twisting or any spinal extension stretching.
Avoid any dancing dips and the limbo dance
which is bad for the spine.

 Avoid any exercise that requires you to be in a
bad uncomfortable postural position.
 Always go easy on any new exercises. Give your
body a chance to get used to them.
Avoid any exercises that require to go beyond the
normal range of a joint. Do not press your luck.
You risk to injure that joint.

Avoid any head stands in yoga positions or other
types of exercises that put a lot of pressure on your
neck and head.. You can easily injure your neck
and the rest of your body if you fall the wrong
way. Your neck is not made to support your whole
body, but just your head.
Avoid any spinal extension exercises especially if
you have scoliosis, it makes the curve worse.

21) HOW TO PREVENT low back injuries and
SCOLIOSIS

There is a saying that "an once of prevention is worth a ton of   therapy."

The best way to prevent scoliosis is exercise , the right exercises that prevents what causes scoliosis which can start as early as soon as a child is born.

By Exercising and avoiding what causes injuries to the joints of your spine and especially the lumbar-sacrum sacroiliac- pelvic joints which is the base and support of the spine , you can prevent low back injuries and scoliosis.
Below is a list of what can cause injuries and scoliosis of the spine. Read and memorized this list and especially learn How to protect your low back from injury that might lead to scoliosis in your every day life.
1) **DO NOT SLEEP ON YOUR STOMACH. Sleeping on your stomach causes strain to your neck and low back and can be the beginning of scoliosis. The best way to sleep is face up and on your side with a small pillow to rest your head on, but not always sleeping on the same side. Sleeping on just one side causes scoliosis and plagiocephaly in kids.
2) DO NOT PLAY ON THE TRAMPOLINE UNLESS YOU HAVE EXPERT TRAINING.**

you can hurt your back and other parts of
your body , from an accidental fall thus
creating the chance of developing scoliosis
 3)NO HEAVY LIFTING AND ALWAYS
BEND YOUR KNEES
When you have to lift anything , even a pencil.

<u>Proper precautions   on how to lift and good
postural habits are essential for all people
whether they have scoliosis or a straight spine,
to protect their spine from injury.</u>

 4)) DO NOT CARRY HEAVY OBJECTS OR
OVERLOADED backpacks and never carry
any objects on one side of your body, because
that forces your spine into a scoliosis curve and
over time it might cause scoliosis.

5) AVOID BAD SITTING POSITIONS ,
When you read , work on the computer, at the
table, at school and especially when you watch
television or movies. Bad sitting positions put a
lot of strain on the sacral -pelvis area and can
cause a lot of health problems including scoliosis
and other postural problems.
6)IF YOU HAVE YOUNGER SIBLINGS OR
NIECES
and nephews do not lift them and never hold

them on one side of your body , as this has the potential to cause strain on your back and eventually scoliosis.

 If you baby-sit younger kids or babies never lift them, that's how most of the girls get their scoliosis.

 7)   Avoid practical jokes and horsing around. Many people had scoliosis and even catastrophic injuries from such practical jokes.

 8) AVOID CONTACT SPORTS like football, wrestling, and hockey.
Many people had lifelong severe injuries to their spine including scoliosis from such sports.

9)AVOID EXCESSIVE HUGGING ,
Especially when your body is in an awkward position and definitely you should Avoid sideways hugs and violent hugs like the " bear hug."
10)if you have to do heavy lifting or work in the garden or anything that has to do with a lot of bending and lifting, use an elastic brace to protect your back. Do as the athletes of heavy lifting do to protect their spines from lifting weights injuries, they use a protective low back belt.

11) if you have pain from strain or sprain in your low back do not ignore it. Use an elastic brace to protect your spine from further injury. If the pain does not go away in a few days see your doctor . By treating an injury early you prevent it from becoming chronic and cause other health problems including scoliosis.

12)   EXERCISE, the last but the most important of all, is to exercise. Exercises are good for any age even for babies. I saw a pediatrician on television giving the mother of a child a prescription... for more exercises for her child. And that's good news. More doctors should give such prescriptions. The right exercises will   make the spine strong, healthy and flexible and when you have strong healthy spinal muscles will protect the spine from any injuries. That's why I designed the   SPINAL ACTIVE FLEXION EXERCISES TO REDUCE IDIOPATHIC SCOLIOSIS in short S.A.F.E.T.R.I.S.
These exercise are good   for prevention of scoliosis by making the spinal muscles strong and the spine healthy and flexible.
These exercises are also very good at correcting any misalignments in the pelvis and spinal joint thus stopping the progression of any abnormal curves in the spine and even reversing it back to

normal.

.

These exercises are designed to make your spine
strong, healthy and more flexible and in the process
to correct any abnormal curves of the spine such as
scoliosis, kyphosis and lordosis. you do not need
any exercise balls or to push your spine one way or
another. these exercises will correct any curve of
the spine by making your spinal muscles strong on
both sides of the spine plus will correct any
misalignment of the pelvic joints which usually is
the mother (the cause) of the scoliosis.... but you
have to do them daily every day for ever.. or at
least when your scoliosis is gone.

22) If you have scoliosis

If you are diagnosed with scoliosis, you should know that you are not alone suffering from this condition. Unfortunately, there are millions of people suffering from this condition. Some of them worse than others. The bigger the Cobb angle is the worse the scoliosis is.
 The most important thing to remember is " that is not your fault." This can happen to anyone at any time for different reasons.
The most important thing you can do is start exercising to stop the progression of the

abnormal curve while it is still small, manageable and can be reversed. The sooner you start the better your chances to reduce the scoliosis while it is still small and manageable. Unfortunately there is no magic pill to take and make the scoliosis disappear .With the spinal exercises you will have a good chance to stop the progression of the abnormal curve and even reverse it back to a healthy spine

Do not expect miracles to happen overnight , but if you have the will, desire and determination to do the exercises daily in the privacy of your home even in your own bed or just a mat on the floor of your house, you will have a good chance to get a strong and healthy spine without any abnormal curve called scoliosis.

If you want to get better and stop the abnormal curve from becoming bigger you have to do the exercises. NOBODY ELSE CAN DO THESE EXERCISES FOR YOU.

IT IS YOUR CHOICE, you do the exercises and you get better or you do nothing and your scoliosis might get worse.

 So far "the wait and see approach" used by many health professionals did not work well for the people suffering from scoliosis and many end up with surgery and rods in their spine.

 If you have pain in your low back along with scoliosis , use an elastic spinal support under

your clothes to protect your spine for any
further injury. Or you can use one of those
corset garment that the women use to wear for
spinal protection and
 Good posture. Of course you remove the

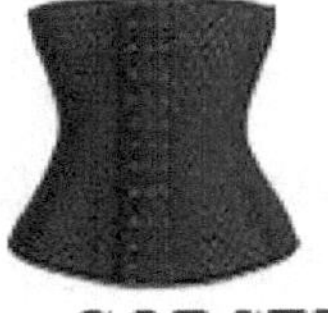

CORSET

support during the exercises.

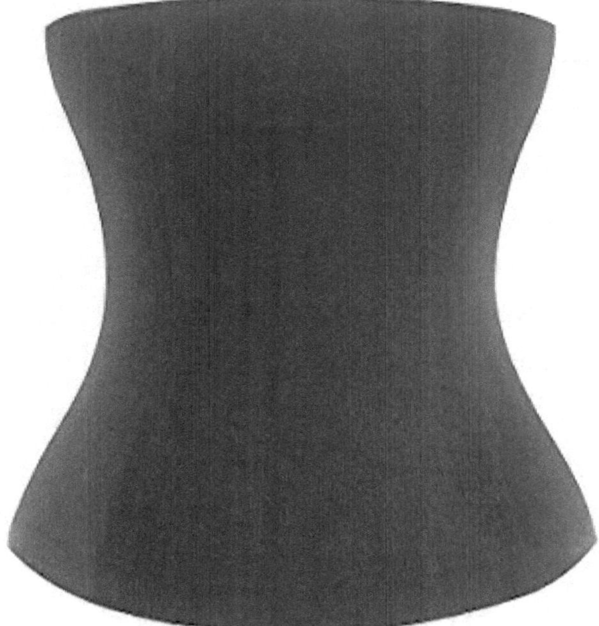

You probably do not need a bulky and expensive
spinal brace.   A fashionable cheap corset might
as well do the same job as an expensive spinal
brace. The idea is to support your spine until
your spine is strong and flexible with the
S.A.F.E.T.R.I.S. exercises you will be doing.

If you decide to use a corset buy one that will give you a good support of your sacroiliac joints and remove it while you exercise .

  There are no guarantees in life, but you will have a good chance to help your self if you have the will, desire and determination to reduce your curve by doing the spinal active flexion exercises daily.

The most important thing to remember is that there is HOPE that the progression of the abnormal spinal curve of your scoliosis can be stopped and even reversed with the right exercises. But you have to have the motivation, the will and determination to exercise daily and avoid any bad postural habits . You and only you can do the exercises and turn your scoliotic spine into a dynamic, healthy, strong and flexible spine without any curves. It is all up to you, take control of your scoliotic spine and turn it to a dynamic strong spine with a perfect posture that will be the envy of many.!
The millions of professional athletes that exercise daily have a perfect posture and a strong healthy spine. You can do it too, with a lot of work, of course, by exercising daily.
Good luck to all of you. I know that you can do it!!

N.B. If the scoliosis is due to pathology or severe trauma ,

or you had surgery with rods in your spine, these exercises are not for you. If that's your case consult your attending doctor for proper treatments and exercise recommendations.

The S.A.F.E.T.R.I.S. exercises are the "ONE STITCH IN TIME TO SAVE NINE" , they have the potential to stop a mild scoliosis(the one stitch) from becoming a severe scoliosis (the nine stitches) requiring, braces and surgery with spinal fusion and rods in the spine . The exercises   will make the spine strong and more flexible without any abnormal curves.

Find the cause of the idiopathic scoliosis   (the lumbar-sacral-pelvic imbalance, malfunction), fix the cause of scoliosis (with the S.A.F.E.T.R.I.S.) or eliminate the cause with the exercises to have strong spinal muscles and a flexible spine without any abnormal curves.

The millions of people that exercise daily prove that exercising   and good nutrition is the

mother of good health and good posture . They have good health ,a strong healthy and flexible spines without any abnormal curves called scoliosis.

23) Conclusion.

The mystery cause of idiopathic scoliosis that baffles the medical and scientific communities and every one else for that matter FROM TIME IMMEMORIAL is, nothing more than an imbalance of the lumbar -sacral-iliac joints . The imbalance of these joints, which is the foundation , the base in which the spinal column sits on it, is the cause of all idiopathic functional and structural scoliosis, "THE MOTHER CAUSE OF SCOLIOSIS"

The x-rays of functional and structural idiopathic scoliosis clearly show the imbalance of those joints with one side of the pelvis, called Ilium , being higher than the other side, the sacrum, as the Greeks call it "the holy bone" which is the base of the spine, tilted to one side.

THE MOTHER CAUSE OF SCOLIOSIS IS PRESENT ON THE X-RAY PICTURES OF EVERY SCOLIOTIC SPINE **BUT HIDING IN CLEAR VIEW** .

 NOW THAT I POINT IT OUT, I HOPE THAT EVERYBODY CAN CLEARLY SEE IT!!

When the foundation of the spine , the sacrum tilts to the side and an imbalance is created, which I name in this book, as "the mother cause of scoliosis" , the spine above has to shift along with the sacrum, thus the scoliosis is starting to form.

 THIS IS THE MOTHER CAUSE OF IDIOPATHIC SCOLIOSIS AND A CROOKED SPINE IS BORN.

In other words the mother cause of scoliosis, or the causative factor of the idiopathic scoliosis is the imbalance of the pelvis-sacral-lumbar joints

caused by a short leg, bad postural habits and strains and injuries to the base of the spine creating the perfect conditions for the development of an initial abnormal curve at the lumbar spine area and a secondary compensatory abnormal curve to the thoracic spine due to the righting reflex trying to bring the centre of gravity within the body's base which are the sacrum and the feet.

The contributing factors to that lumbar-sacrum-iliac imbalance are the anatomical short leg, bad postural habits and injuries and strains of the low back.
When we eliminate the above contributing factors to the lumbar-sacrum-iliac imbalance, and with the .S.A.F.E.T.R.I.S. EXERCISES that imbalance and malfunction of those joints should return to normal and the abnormal spinal curve will go away the same way that it was created.

It is my hope that this revelation of the "mother cause of scoliosis" will result in better and faster treatments for the so called idiopathic scoliosis, now that we know both the cause, and the contributing factors to that lumbar-sacrum- iliac imbalance. It should be early diagnosis and early treatments   with the S.A.F.E.T.R.I.IS. Exercises and the use of sacroiliac support if needed, without any delays, correcting a small functional spinal curve before it becomes a huge structural curve and a life long suffering.

24) Epilogue

I always wanted to write about scoliosis but it was not easy to find a suitable publisher to publish a book.
Thanks to the self-publishing of the Amazon Kindle direct Publishing I am finally able to publish my books.
It is not important how many people buy my books, or how much money I make from my books.
People do not write books to make money, at least I do not, but people write books from time immemorial in order to convey knowledge and other people benefit from that knowledge in the books.
The important thing is that I am able to publish my books and   are available as eBooks and in

print for anybody to read them and benefit from
what I write in my books..
My life long quest to find out what is the cause of
scoliosis and how to prevent and treat it , is
finally achieved and it is written down in books
for anyone to read them and benefit from my
writings.
As with anything else, there is no guarantee that
everyone that reads my books will benefit from
them, but no matter what percentage of people
with scoliosis will benefit and stop the
progression of their abnormal spinal curve and
even reverse it, it is still a number of people that
will definitely benefit and have a better life with a
strong, healthy and flexible spine, because of
reading my books.
 And that's the most gratifying feeling knowing
that my writings contributed to some people to
have a better quality of life !
I know that there are going to be some skeptics
and nonbelievers that might criticize the way I
see the **mother- cause** of idiopathic scoliosis and
the recommended treatments with the spinal
active flexion exercises to reduce idiopathic
scoliosis in short S.A.F.E.T.R.I.S. but that's ok
with me. At least, it will start the conversation
about the cause of idiopathic scoliosis and the
existing treatments and the quest for better
treatments without any delay. The so called

OBSERVATION PERIOD , definitely does not
serve the needs of the people with scoliosis, and
they waste a lot of precious time while a small
functional spinal curve, which could easily be
stopped and even reversed, becomes a severe
structural curve requiring surgery and rods in the
spine.
If anyone else out there has a better explanation
about the cause of idiopathic scoliosis and any
contributing factors other than the ones that I
describe, I will be more than happy to look at it.
As a matter of fact I will be excited and very
happy, if someone else has a better   explanation
about the cause of scoliosis and better exercises
that reverse the spinal curve in a shorter period of
time .   And above all never dismiss anything
before you try it.   Whether you have scoliosis or
not, go ahead ,try exercising daily with the spinal
active flexion exercises and see for yourself how
much better you will feel.
  But please do not tell me about abstract theories
developed in a sterile laboratory, or in the figment
of someone's vivid imagination. I happen to like
facts and not theories.
**<u>The mother cause of scoliosis, the lumbar-
sacrum-iliac imbalance</u>** is hiding in clear view in
the x-ray pictures of every idiopathic scoliosis.
All you have to do is just look at the x-ray , after
x-ray of scoliotic spines of every age, and I am

sure you will clearly see it, now that I point it out for everyone to see.

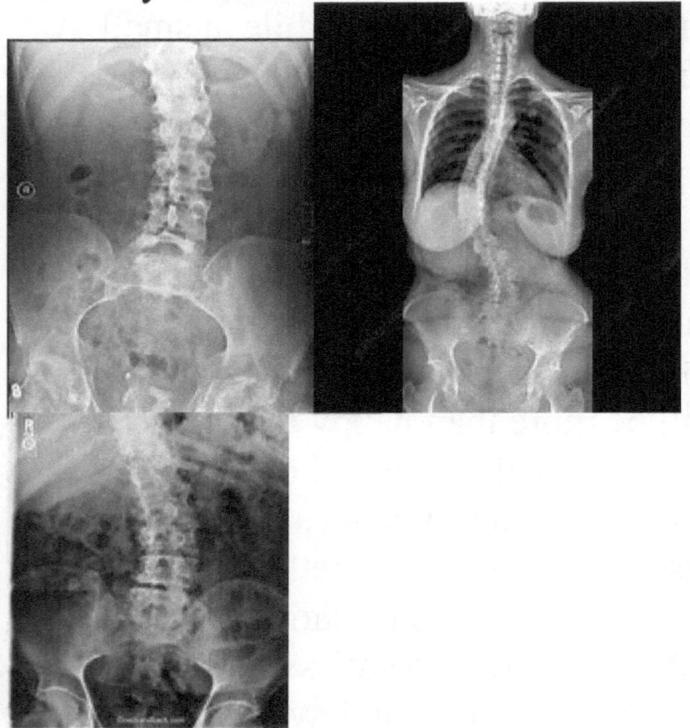

To all the people that suffer with scoliosis I wish you all good luck and speedy reversal of your abnormal spinal curve ,with the exercises S.A.F.E.T.R.I.S. Take control of your scoliotic spine ,   eliminate any bad postural habits and with hard work exercising daily there is hope to turn your spine into a strong healthy and flexible spine with a good posture that will be the envy of many! The spine is the backbone of good health , good posture and splendor .The secret to keep your spine healthy, strong and flexible is to exercise daily.

With the S.A.F.E.T.R.I.S. exercises you do not
have to go to the gym or buy any expensive
equipment . All you need is your motivation,
your will, your determination and the desire to get
better by exercising daily.
.

It is my sincere hope that all the people that do
the SPINAL ACTIVE FLEXION EXERCISES
TO REDUCE THE IDIOPATHIC SCOLIOSIS
daily, will get what they were looking for to
reduce their scoliosis and in the process have a
strong , healthy, flexible spine , and good posture
with no abnormal spinal curves.

It is also my hope that this book will start the
conversation for the prevention and better
treatments for people diagnosed with idiopathic
scoliosis.
Idiopathic scoliosis is a preventable and treatable
condition   and the key for a strong ,healthy and
flexible spine without any abnormal curves is the
right spinal exercises!
Exercises is the key for good health, good posture
and   a sharp mind!
The ancient Greeks used to say "νους υγιης εν
σωματι υγιη», a healthy mind in a healthy body.

Good luck to all, and I wish everybody   to have a

sharp mind and a strong healthy body without any abnormal spinal curves.

DR. S. ELIA

25) References

1) congenital scoliosis cause:" Jan 26, 2007Allen J. Wilcox, M.D., Ph.D., lead NIEHS author on the new study published online in the *British Medical Journal.* "

 2) **A Dangerous Curve: The Role of History in America's Scoliosis Screening Programs**

3) **ADAMS TEST**

4) **x-ray pictures courtesy of " images of free X-ray pictures of idiopathic scoliosis from the internet by bing.com/images**

5) **A FRESH LOOK AT WHAT CAUSES THE IDIOPATHIC FUNCTIONAL SCOLIOSIS AND HOME EXERCISES TO STOP THE PROGRESSION OF THE CURVE AND EVEN REVERSE IT BACK TO NORMAL By S.ELIA**

6)GIRLS' SCOLIOSIS by S. ELIA

26) For the cover book

Idiopathic scoliosis is a preventable and treatable condition.
The quest that baffles the medical and scientific communities from time immemorial, what is causing the idiopathic scoliosis, is finally answered.
Read this book to find out the answer to that million dollar question!

In this book you will find what is the real cause of the abnormal curve called scoliosis.
In this book you will find the mother cause of scoliosis.
Read this book to find out the contributing   factors to the mother cause of scoliosis.
The million dollar question that baffles the medical and scientific community ever since the father of medicine HIPPOCRATES named the crooked spine scoliosis, is finally answered, and graphically explained!
If you have scoliosis this book will tell you what is causing your scoliosis and ways to stop the progression of that abnormal curve.
.

If you contemplating to have healthy kids, read this book to see what vitamin is essential to prevent congenital scoliosis, spinal bifida, cleft lips and cleft palate.
If your child is diagnosed with scoliosis read this book to find the causative factors of the idiopathic scoliosis and what exercises to do to stop the progression of the abnormal curve..
Finally read this book just out of curiosity to find out what is the real" mother cause of the idiopathic scoliosis" that baffles the medical and scientific community from time immemorial.

27)From the inside cover:

After you read this book and you no longer need it , give it to someone else to read and benefit from the knowledge in this book.
Knowledge is to be shared for the benefit all.

Other books published by the same author.

1)ALZHEIMER'S AND DEMENTIA:HOW TO REDUCE THE RISKS OF ALZHEIMER'S AND WAYS TO IMPROVE THE QUALITY OF LIFE: WHY SOME PEOPLE LIVE A LONG HEALTHY LIFE AND OTHERS GET ALZHEIMER'S
Paperback
- **ASIN:** 1090253281
- **ISBN-13:** 978-1090253286

© 2018 BY S. ELIA ALL RIGHTS RESERVED

2)AN ANTHOLOGY OF GREEK AND ENGLISH POEMS AND SONGS:
ΕΛΛΗΝΙΚΑ ΚΑΙ ΑΓΛΙΚΑ ΠΟΙΗΜΑΤΑ ΚΑΙ ΤΡΑΓΟΥΔΙΑ
Paperback
- **ASIN:** 1790886384
- **ISBN-13:** 978-1790886388

© 2018 BY S.ELIA all rights reserved

3)CONSTIPATION:HOW TO PREVENT AND TREAT CONSTIPATION: DIET IS THE KEY FOR PREVENTING CONSTIPATION

Paperback

- **ASIN:** 1091554803
- **ISBN-13:** 978-1091554801

4)EAT THE RIGHT FOODS FOR OPTIMUM HEALTH :: These nutritional foods are reasonably priced for any budget.
Paperback

- **ASIN:** 1796857157
- **ISBN-13:** 978-1796857153

5)GIRLS' SCOLIOSIS:WHY MORE GIRLS ARE AFFECTED THAN BOYS? THE CAUSE, PREVENTION AND TREATMENTS: ~TAKE CARE OF YOUR SPINE, IT IS THE BACKBONE OF GOOD HEALTH, BEARING AND SPLENDOR
Paperback

- **ASIN:** 1072357461
- **ISBN-13:** 978-1072357469

6)HOME EXERCISES FOR GOOD POSTURE:Good posture means good looks and good health: Best Exercises for good posture in the privacy of your own home.
Paperback

- **ASIN:** 1798573997
- **ISBN-13:** 978-1798573990

- 7)my poems and songs: original lyrics

Paperback

- **ASIN:** 1729055397
- **ISBN-13:** 978-1729055397

8) THE PROS AND CONS OF THE HUMAN HUG: STOP THAT DANGEROUS HUG BEFORE IT RUINS YOUR HEALTH AND OR YOUR FEELINGS.
Paperback

- **ASIN:** 1731523955
- **ISBN-13:** 978-1731523952

9)SCOLIOSIS:: A FRESH LOOK AT WHAT CAUSES THE IDIOPATHIC FUNCTIONAL SCOLIOSIS AND HOME EXERCISES TO STOP THE PROGRESSION OF THE CURVE AND EVEN REVERSE IT BACK TO NORMAL
Paperback

- **ASIN:** 1726772233
- **ISBN-13:** 978-1726772235

10) SCOLIOSIS: HOW TO PREVENT AND TREAT SCOLIOSIS WITH THE SPINAL ACTIVE FLEXION EXERCISES (S.A.F.E.)
Paperback

- **ASIN:** 1728674816
- **ISBN-13:** 978-1728674810

11)SCOLIOSIS:: A FRESH LOOK AT WHAT CAUSES THE IDIOPATHIC FUNCTIONAL SCOLIOSIS AND HOME EXERCISES TO STOP THE PROGRESSION OF THE CURVE AND EVEN REVERSE IT BACK TO NORMAL
Paperback

- **ASIN:** 1790493161
- **ISBN-13:** 978-1790493166

12)TAKE CONTROL OF YOUR SCOLIOSIS: ONLY YOU CAN TURN YOUR SCOLIOTIC SPINE INTO A DYNAMIC, STRONG, HEALTHY AND FLEXIBLE SPINE WITH THE HOME SPINAL ACTIVE FLEXION EXERCISES(S.A.F.E.)
Paperback

- **ASIN:** 1730978797
- **ISBN-13:** 978-1730978791

28)From the author.
It is my sincere hope ,that everybody that reads this
book and exercises daily with the S.A.F.E.T.R.I.S.
EXERCISES, will   turn their spine into a strong,
healthy and dynamic spine without any abnormal
curves and in the process they get good health and
a posture that will be the envy of many!
Spread the word that there is hope to stop the
progression and even reverse it back to normal, of
that abnormal spinal curve, called scoliosis .

Dr. s. elia